Number Training Your Brain

Number Training Your Brain

Jonathan Hancock and
Jon Chapman

Hodder Education

338 Euston Road, London NW1 3BH.

Hodder Education is an Hachette UK company

First published in UK 2011 by Hodder Education

First published in US 2011 by The McGraw-Hill Companies, Inc.

This edition published 2011.

10 9 8 7 6 5 4 3 2 1

The publisher has used its best endeavours to ensure that any website addresses referred to in this book are correct and active at the time of going to press. However, the publisher and the author have no responsibility for the websites and can make no guarantee that a site will remain live or that the content will remain relevant, decent or appropriate.

The publisher has made every effort to mark as such all words which it believes to be trademarks. The publisher should also like to make it clear that the presence of a word in the book, whether marked or unmarked, in no way affects its legal status as a trademark.

Every reasonable effort has been made by the publisher to trace the copyright holders of material in this book. Any errors or omissions should be notified in writing to the publisher, who will endeavour to rectify the situation for any reprints and future editions.

Hachette UK's policy is to use papers that are natural, renewable and recyclable products and made from wood grown in sustainable forests. The logging and manufacturing processes are expected to conform to the environmental regulations of the country of origin.

www.hoddereducation.co.uk

Typeset by MPS Limited, a Macmillan Company.

Printed in Great Britain by CPI Cox & Wyman, Reading.

Acknowledgements

We'd like to thank Victoria Roddam and her team at Hodder for the support given to this book at every stage.

Thank you also to our agent, Caroline Shott, and to everyone at The Learning Skills Foundation.

We're very grateful to our families for their patience while we juggled our 'real-life' commitments and put this book together from both sides of the world.

A number of relatives, friends and colleagues gave us useful feedback along the way. Particular thanks go to Andrew Clingan and Richard Hancock. We've appreciated their careful reading and helpful comments, but any mistakes that remain are ours!

Image credits

Contents

Meet the authors

Welcome to the world of number training: a place where your mental muscles will be flexed like never before. Get ready to take your thinking skills in some exciting new directions and to feel better than ever about the strength of your brain.

To us – a brain trainer and a maths professor – 'number training' means building up your brain power to get the most out of mathematical thinking. By exploring the rich universe of maths, mastering some key techniques and getting a feel for the way the best mathematicians' minds work, we're confident that you can learn ways of using your own brain better. The thinking tricks you collect here will equip you to cope with more of the maths life throws your way, but they'll also boost your overall mental strength and agility and give you an edge in many different sorts of challenge.

Put simply, we think it's good for your brain to think about maths. We want to show you that numbers can delight, divert, but also *develop* your thinking. When you know how to find and exploit them, the opportunities to train your brain with numbers are infinite (and infinity is just one of the challenging concepts your maths mind is about to tackle).

So, whatever your previous experience has been, we think you'll be surprised by just how good your mathematical thinking can be now – and how much it can add to your life. We hope our book entertains, surprises, challenges and inspires, and takes you that bit closer to your goal of having a well-trained brain.

In one minute

Number training helps you to use your brain better.
It's healthy, useful, impressive, fun… and to prove it:

Hand your friend a calculator – and, as you do so,
secretly spot a number between 1 and 100 somewhere in
the room.

> ▶ *Number training will get you noticing and exploring*
> *numbers wherever they appear.*

Ask your friend to say any three-digit number and
to enter it into the calculator. Then, to multiply it by ten,
subtract their number, divide this result *by* their number,
square the answer, and add 19.

> ▶ *Number training will help you to explain these*
> *processes clearly, and to give all the instructions*
> *from memory.*

Now secretly, *mentally*, subtract your secret number
from 100.

> ▶ *Number training will sharpen all your calculating*
> *skills.*

Whatever answer you get, tell your friend to take this
number away from the running total. Then, just as they
hit the equals key, go over to your number, point to it, and
listen out for a gasp of astonishment as the same number
appears on the calculator screen.

> ▶ *Number training will take your mental confidence to*
> *a whole new level.*

Exploring numbers reveals powerful ways to use your
brain, stretching your thinking skills in every direction and
activating some truly impressive abilities. Prepare to amaze
yourself with what you can do. When you know how
to make the most of it, maths can be mind-bending and
magical.

Introduction to number training

We used to think that our brains simply faded away, the precious cells disappearing inevitably over time, like sand through an hourglass. The life-story of the brain was pretty depressing – until, in recent years, neuroscience began to paint a much rosier picture. The human brain was revealed to be 'plastic': still undergoing a great deal of change over a lifetime, due to environment and experience, but capable of changing for the better. The big news was that key areas could be physically strengthened by the way they're used. Suddenly we realized it was possible for us to rewire our brains to match our needs, boosting processing power and extending thinking skills. It was a thrilling idea, and the basis for the whole brain-training revolution.

But can the puzzles and exercises in books, newspapers and computer games really 'train your brain' as a whole – or do they just improve your skills at those particular challenges? Will brain training ever have any real impact on areas of thought that you *haven't* practised? Initial claims about the wide-reaching benefits of brain training – especially this very attractive promise of general improvement, or 'far transfer' – have been thrown into question recently by a number of studies. Doing Sudoku puzzles, crosswords or logic problems certainly makes you better at those things, but whether or not they help you improve in other tasks – even those that share some of the same elements – is unclear.

So, while there's good evidence about active minds staying active for longer, and even fending off the symptoms of some degenerative conditions, we just don't know yet if training really can build a better brain overall. But we're still very confident about the benefits of number training because our approach capitalizes on all the good news from neuroscience: the bits that have been proved beyond doubt.

Practising certain thinking tasks makes you better at them, and can strengthen those particular bits of your brain, so it makes good sense to stretch your mental muscles in every direction imaginable and to develop the widest possible repertoire of skills. Maths offers such a huge range of challenges, with all the key thinking strategies involved in a rich mix of connections and combinations. The puzzles, games and exercises in this book are designed to give your brain a full workout and to help you bring together all the core mental habits necessary for success. Crucially, to *keep* you practising them, we think the brain-training tasks you choose need to be interesting, stimulating, motivating and inspiring.

Repeating easy calculations at speed may be useful mental exercise, and there are plenty of books and games on the market that will provide you with long lists of questions. You can time yourself, improve your speed and accuracy, and help to keep your basic calculation skills sharp. But we know that number training can go further than that – and *needs* to, if you're going to stay with it and enjoy the wide-ranging benefits on offer. There's so much more to maths than simple sums.

▶ 28 is a 'perfect number' – equal to the sum of all its factors: $1 + 2 + 4 + 7 + 14 = 28$.
▶ Each of the first ten square numbers is the sum of consecutive odd numbers: for example, 4 (which is 2×2) is the sum of 1 and 3; 81 (or 9×9) is equal to $1 + 3 + 5 \ldots + 17$.
▶ A number is only divisible by 9 if its digit-sum is too.
▶ If A is 1, B is 2 and so on, the letters in the word 'numeracy' add up to exactly 100!

Check these four facts in your head now and you're already beginning to stretch some key mental muscles. We want this book to demonstrate the fun you can have with maths when you start learning its secrets and tricks. We include examples from the lives of history's greatest mathematical minds, stories of long-held obsessions with theorems and conjectures, and thinking challenges that will keep you interested and inspire you to push your brain towards new levels of agility, focus and understanding.

At its best, brain training gives you a real sense of mental wellbeing. You develop new skills, improve your speed and accuracy and *feel* your brain changing to support your ongoing progress. But you also start to appreciate the benefits in some very practical ways. We want to show you how numbers can explain, simplify, solve, accelerate and improve many aspects of everyday life. With a little guidance, you'll soon see that maths offers brain-training challenges everywhere you look: opportunities to put your understanding to good use, to build your core thinking skills and keep your brain flexible and sharp.

We'll show you quick calculation methods to help you get the best shopping deals, techniques for assessing betting odds under pressure, tricks for manipulating numbers to entertain and amaze, strategies for pushing logic to its limits... and underlying all these systems and skills are thinking habits that you can definitely transfer to other tasks – because we'll show you how.

You may need to brush up on a few aspects of maths to start putting these training methods to use – but don't worry, numbers don't really come naturally to *anyone*.

They're a human invention, based on natural instincts to count and calculate and understand, but are really just the agreed ways of operating and communicating that we all have to learn. The things you try to do with numbers may be instinctive, but the numbers themselves need to be made to work for you – which is powerful brain training in itself, forcing you to grapple with symbols and systems. You exercise memory, visualization and logic; and, as you start to use the processes, your maths work pushes you to be more creative, to make decisions in new ways, to notice details, recognize patterns, connect different areas of thought, and achieve a brain capable of making not just calculations but *conclusions*.

Part one explores the important things you need to know about numbers. We explain the system, show you how to work it, and reveal why it can provide such a great workout for your brain.

Part two takes you on a whistle-stop tour of the wider world of maths, picking out areas of interest and challenge wherever they occur: in geometry, algebra, data-handling... It explains how mathematicians' minds are constantly being stretched by the biggest questions, and explores how your brain can be improved by employing mathematical thinking skills in your own daily life.

The great French philosopher and mathematician Rene Descartes stressed that maths was much more than a particular field of 'numerical science'. To him, thinking mathematically offered great chances to learn the truth in all the other fields of enquiry – using all the thinking skills at work in a trained brain. He saw the importance of numbers in fields like music, mechanics and astronomy, noticing that they all relied on sequence and measurement that could be explored using mathematical thought. To Descartes, maths was about reasoning, using an agreed, planned language to deliver answers. (So he would have been delighted by all the scientific discoveries made in the twentieth century that had been predicted many years earlier by mathematical minds.)

But what would he have made of our modern-day reliance on technology to do so much of the maths for us? Now that mobile phones can be used to do complex calculations, and supercomputers are testing theories in ways that no human brain can manage, will our mathematical thinking fall by the wayside? Then again, maybe we're just being released from all the boring bits, the mechanical calculating, and freed to use our mathematical brains in new and exciting ways.

In this book we explore how maths can sharpen your thinking skills, showing why it's still important to have the key techniques at your fingertips. But times change, brains change, and the most exciting possibilities for us lie in what a number-trained brain can achieve today, going beyond individual calculations to achieve new levels of mental fitness and finding original and intriguing applications for mathematical thought.

Number training puts the ball firmly in your court. A baby's brain cells may have more interconnections than an adult's, but your older model has been customized to work in particular ways, its key areas developed and enhanced, and that process can continue throughout your life. Pioneer of brain research Wilder Penfield showed that an individual's thinking processes become mapped out in different designs, reflecting their unique experiences and needs. Musicians, for example, have more processing capacity relating to the body parts they use the most. Their mental maps for pitch and tone are bigger, the neurons better adapted to differentiating between sounds. Your brain is constantly adapting to the way you use it – so you'd better be using it well!

Training your brain with maths may lead to some helpful changes in your physical brain, but it will certainly sharpen a range of mental areas, including many of the abilities valued by traditional tests of intelligence – such as pattern-finding, code-breaking, orientation and reasoning. Rather than being about how far you went in your education, and the particular systems you may or may not have understood at school, being *really* good at maths involves visualization, memory, creative thinking... a repertoire of key thinking skills that can have a major impact on all the challenges you turn your mind to.

And at last our education system is catching on. There's a new emphasis in schools on mental maths, plus a commitment to teaching the core mathematical thinking skills, rather than just particular systems of calculation. Countries that delay the use of written methods are reporting impressive results, one theory being that their children are less bound by the 'rules' and more able to choose creatively from a range of possible approaches. It's a crucial ability to have. Have a go at the following three calculations in your head:

$$12 + 35 \qquad\qquad 39 + 17 \qquad\qquad 99 + 98$$

Three straightforward sums – but you may well have found yourself using three different calculating strategies. (The answers, by the way, are 47, 56 and 197.) Developing your mental flexibility is a key goal of number training. We hope you'll strengthen your understanding of the maths itself along the way, but even more important is your ability to choose from all the strategies at your disposal. With practice, you'll become more aware of the relationships between numbers, able to spot patterns and parallels, to make clever choices about pursuing answers, and then to use them in the most effective ways.

A trained brain sees the interconnections between many different aspects of maths. Each chapter in the book focuses on one particular area of mathematical thought, but there's also an ongoing theme about the need to break down barriers and to see where ideas intersect. We hope these new connections will themselves expand your thinking, providing a glimpse of the real beauty of maths as well as an awareness of its powerful presence in the world around you.

From a product's design to its supermarket barcode, from road layout to traffic-light sequencing, maths is woven into the fabric of daily life. It's embedded in our language – 'the third degree', 'at sixes and sevens', 'the whole nine yards'. Mathematics has influenced architecture and art through the ages. The famous 'Golden Number', 1.618, known about more than 2,000 years ago, was used to design Ancient Greek temples and to help artists like Leonardo da Vinci and Piet Mondrian proportion their paintings. The musical scale can be understood as a clear number sequence. Mathematical order is even apparent in the workings of nature. Fibonacci's famous sequence

0, 1, 1, 2, 3, 5, 8, 13 … (where each number is the sum of the previous two) is seen clearly in the arrangement of seeds on flower heads and the proportions of shell spirals. Cicadas rely on prime numbers to keep their population cycles out of synch with their predators. There are patterns in nature, revealed by maths, and number training will give you new ways to explore the world, to see beauty in its design, and to stretch all your thinking skills as you investigate maths wherever and whenever it appears.

We want to free you from any fears you might have about maths, so prepare to take a break from some of the written techniques you learned – or tried to learn – at school. Make sure you don't miss all the opportunities to develop the really important aspects of your mathematical thinking.

Visualization

Question 1: If you attach a string to the corner of an ice-cube and dangle it in a glass of water so that half of it is getting wet, what shape does it make in the water when you look down from above? (Don't worry if you don't get this one straight away; it's hard, but you can do it!)

Question 2: What number is below the 3 on your mobile phone keypad?

Question 3: How many different ways can you replace the drawer of a matchbox?

Number training will improve your ability to visualize: numbers, shapes, movement, pattern… and to pick out the key elements in any question you face. You'll understand more about what you're being asked and have new ways to manipulate information on the way to finding the answer.

Memory

The first 20 digits of Pi are 3.1415926535897932384. Give yourself two minutes to memorize them, using any technique that works for you, then cover the numbers and see if you can read them out from memory, in sequence, then in reverse order. What's the ninth digit after the decimal point? Which three numbers come before 323?

Question 4: Start with 1. Add 17. Divide by 3. Multiply by 2. Add 49. Subtract the number you started with. Divide by 4. Divide by 2. Multiply by 1,000. Add the number of days in March. Whatever number you have in your head now, add together all the digits. Find the square root, then divide by 4. What number do you get at the end?

At various points in the book, we explore the importance of memory in maths: remembering important numbers, recalling times tables, memorizing useful techniques and tricks, and using memory strategies to hold digits in your head through all the steps of a mental calculation. Maths relies on memory – and many of the puzzles and exercises in this book provide excellent opportunities for keeping your memory skills sharp.

The 'extended mind'

This is a recurring theme in number training: the idea of using and incorporating the physical world in mental calculations. It links to kinaesthetic learning – learning by doing – but takes it a stage further. The aim is to use the body and environment to provide frameworks for thinking that can become internalized – 'built into' the brain.

Author insight: Jon

I leave my keys by the front door to help me remember them. The place where they live is almost an extension of my memory. I use the shape of objects around me to solve geometry questions. I may be a maths professor but I still hold up my fingers sometimes to help me count. There are many ways to strengthen and extend your thinking by connecting it to your body, your location, and all the useful props available. We've been extending our minds in this way for thousands of years; in fact, it's helped us develop many of our most important number systems, so it makes sense to use anything we can to structure and support our thinking.

Focused thinking

Maths helps you train your brain to identify the key facts in any sort of problem. You'll get better at separating the important bits from the red-herrings, intellect from emotion, and learn to recognize the habits of thought that can skew your understanding and wreck your calculations.

Logic

Maths is logical, and mathematical thinking is about making an argument that stands up to rigorous testing.

Creativity

How could you use a 30 cm ruler to measure the height of a tower block? You might divide the building into small sections and then use multiplication to find the total. What if you stood far back enough for the tower block to be exactly hidden behind the ruler: would that tell you anything? Perhaps you could do something with shadows, or the time it took for the ruler to fall if you threw it from the top floor – or simply offer the ruler as a bribe to the building's owner to tell you the answer.

Logic is central to number training, but there's still plenty of room for creativity. This book explores some famous questions that have, so far, resisted all logic – including the processing power of supercomputers – and may well require a creative approach if they're to be beaten. Creative calculating can save time, unearth new maths applications, and extend your thinking skills to solve other sorts of problems in original ways.

> **Authors' insight**
>
> To solve Fermat's infamous 'Last Theorem', mathematician Andrew Wiles had to borrow creatively from many different areas of maths. Other great maths minds have combined ideas and made surprising connections, gaining inspiration from unlikely places and demonstrating yet more useful thinking habits obtained from the practice of maths.

Every aspect of your maths will be boosted by honing visualization, strengthening memory, using your environment, focusing on facts, trusting logic, expanding creativity… and finding flexible ways to combine these valuable thinking skills. Crucially, these are all skills that can be applied to a range of other challenges in life, generating benefits at every turn, boosting overall mental confidence, and helping you to set up your brain for the success it deserves.

Throughout the book you'll be meeting characters from different times and places who exemplify these attributes. Look out for the 'Names in numbers' feature because these people all have important lessons to pass on: about how to do maths, and about how to push mathematical thinking to the limit.

Within every chapter there are questions to stretch your thinking skills, plus a test at the end: ten maths challenges based on key themes from the chapter along with ideas to keep practising from earlier in the book.

But before you start your training…

Test yourself now

Use the following questions to assess your existing abilities. Do your best with each section, check your answers, and keep a note of your performance: how well you do, but also how good you feel about your skills. You'll be taking a similar set of tests at the end of the book to help you gauge just how far you've come.

VISUALIZATION

Question 1: You have six matches. How can you arrange them to make four equilateral triangles?

Question 2: Without rotating the page, what would the following sequences of numbers and letters look like upside down?

a) 96Npq   b) 806sHb9   c) 9Xd60W86q

Question 3: How many capital letters have at least one line of symmetry?

Question 4: You leave your friend's house and travel due north, turning right at the traffic lights. You drive in that direction for a few minutes before turning left, right and right again. The road takes you under the railway bridge, then you take a sharp right at the church – at which point you realize you've gone wrong, do a 180 degree turn, drive in that direction as far as the museum and turn left into the road where your daughter's at a birthday party. Assuming that this and all the other roads are straight, which way is your car facing now?

MEMORY

Question 5: Spend one minute memorizing the following grid of numbers.

1	8	6	4
7	9	3	2
2	1	7	4
7	2	8	0

Now cover the grid and answer these questions from memory:

a) What are the digits in the four corners of the grid?
b) How many sevens are there?
c) Which number is above the nine?
d) What's the total of the four central digits?

Question 6: Carry out the following five calculations, in order, from memory. Then, work out the letter values of your answers (if 1 = A, 2 = B, etc.) to reveal an appropriate word. Your challenge is to carry out this whole task in your head.

a) 25 × 3	− 7	÷ 2	+ 14	÷ 2	− 22
b) 1,000 ÷ 50	× 3	− 48	÷ 4	× 7	− 3
c) 3,620 ÷ 10	+ 18	÷ 2	− 69	÷ 11	− 10
d) 6 × 40	+ 10	× 5	− 333	× 2	− 1,825
e) 3 × 7	+ 47	× 2	+ 4	÷ 5	÷ 2

Question 7: You have one minute to study the shape below.

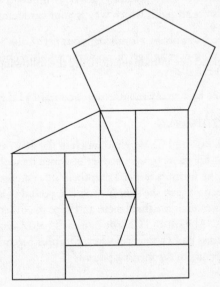

Make sure you can't see the illustration as you answer the following questions from memory.

a) How many rectangles appeared in the picture you saw?
b) How many triangles were there?
c) What was the total number of diagonal lines?

EXTENDED MIND

Teach yourself (or revise, if you were shown it at school) the following finger trick to work out the number of days in each calendar month.

Make a fist with one of your hands so that you can see the knuckles of four fingers and the spaces between them. Count through the months in order, touching the first knuckle when you say January, the space next to it for February, the next knuckle on March, and so on – until you mark July on the index finger knuckle. Then go back to the first knuckle for August and continue as before. The significance of this odd-looking activity is that every knuckle represents a month that has 31 days.

Question 8: Now put this technique to the test by working out whether or not the following months have 31 days:

a) March
b) October
c) June

And can you do it simply by *visualizing* your fist? Look at your real fist, then close your eyes and go through the whole month-counting process in your mind's eye.

d) Can you say how many months *don't* contain 31 days?

FOCUSED THINKING

Question 9: Al, Bob and Charlie had lunch in the new cafe on the high street. The bill came to £30, so all three men handed over a £10 note. But then the waitress noticed that there'd been mistake. The bill should have been £25; so she simply took five pound coins out of the till, gave one to each of the three men, and kept the other two coins for herself. So... Al, Bob and Charlie had each paid £9, or £27 in total. The waitress had £2 in her pocket. £27 plus £2 comes to £29. So what's happened to the missing pound?

LOGIC

Question 10: Cannibals caught three explorers as they trekked through the jungle. They told the men they were going to be eaten, unless they could solve a puzzle. The men would have just one chance to avoid being dinner.

The cannibals lined up the men and tied each of them to a stake. The first man could see the backs of the other two. The one in the middle could see his friend in front. The man at the front wasn't able to see anyone. The three men were then shown five tribal hats: three covered in black fur, the other two white. Each of the men was blindfolded for a moment while a hat was placed on his head and the two spare hats taken away. Finally the blindfolds were removed and the men were told that, in less than a minute, one of them had to work out the colour of his own hat – or it would be dinner-time…

The man at the back said quickly, 'I don't know.' The one in the middle spoke next: 'I don't know either.' But the man at the front smiled. 'I know,' he said.

How did he do it – and what colour was his hat?

CREATIVITY

Question 11: Look carefully at this L-shaped arrangement of coins:

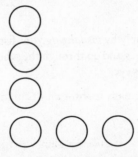

We want there to be four coins in the vertical line and four in the horizontal line. How can you do that – by moving only one coin?

Question 12: Draw one line into the following equation to make it correct:

5 + 5 + 5 = 550

Question 13: When does 11 + 2 = 1?

To check your answers, go to the Answers section at the back of the book.

Part one

Thinking about numbers

1

Mathematical minds: the story so far

In this chapter you will learn:
- *about the human instinct to count and calculate*
- *the history of number systems*
- *why place value is so important, and the benefits of going beyond base ten*
- *exercises and games to explore key mental maths techniques.*

The numbers of nature

In the curves of rivers, the arrangement of flower petals, the patterns of populations, there's mathematical order in nature. We respond to this order when we see it, we try to create it when we don't, and we seem to have a natural urge to quantify, organize and understand the world with numbers.

We're not the only animals who can count. Crows and magpies, for example, never raid nests where there are four or fewer eggs, because the owner will quickly spot that there's one missing. A chimpanzee called Amyumu trounced memory expert Ben Pridmore in a test that involved recalling and ordering sets of numbers on a computer screen.

THE BIRTH OF NUMBER THINKING

In humans, counting skills start developing even before birth. Scientists found that babies who were played number rhythms in the womb were better at recognizing and responding to them in the outside world. Anyone who's spent time with young children will know the fascination they feel for counting – toys, cars, stairs, anything – as they begin to learn how things work and look for ways to describe what they discover. It's no wonder that so many songs and rhymes are based on numbers and simple sequences, making the most of the comforting regularity of numbers, and our in-built urge to count.

There's evidence that children need no teaching to learn about one, two, three and four, but stop there. We're good at recognizing up to four distinct things, but beyond that our brains seem to hit a barrier. Four is as far as egg-stealing birds go; but humans too have problems going further, without help. Psychologists call it the difference between 'subitizing' and counting. We can subitize up to four items in a quarter of a second, but then we need a whole second to count every four items after that.

The Botocudos, nomadic hunter-gatherers from the Brazilian rainforest, only had words for the numbers one and two, pushed on to three and four by using them in combination (three made up from two and one, four from two and two), but could go no further until they developed a system of body counting. They worked out patterns of touching fingers, wrists, necks – excellent 'extended mind' thinking – and then could check and compare amounts by running back through these agreed sequences. The ancient Romans only chose names for their first four sons before relying on numbers: Quintus, Sextus, Septimus… Of course the Romans also developed the ancient tradition of tallying, leaving their own mark on the history of counting, but their calendar only had four 'proper' names for months before a numbering process took over again: Quintilis, Sextilis, September… Like the rest of us, their brains needed systematic help.

We have evidence of counting systems being used more than 30,000 years ago. At different times and locations they have been developed to suit particular needs for numbers, but there are some key themes in the varied methods agreed: like tally marks to speed up recording and counting; things from the physical world brought in to augment brain power; and a few digits employed to represent all the numbers required. These are all important aspects of the way we count today, reflecting some of the fundamental workings of our mathematical minds.

Tallying

Our word 'tally' comes from the same place as 'tailor', describing the ancient art of cutting marks to record numbers. From one-to-one tallying to the typical groups of five marks used today – via Roman numerals, just an extension of tallying – the system has been developed and refined.

Try these tallying tests below. How quickly can you count the following marks? Have a go at each set, touching the page if necessary, but also trying to do it with your eyes alone. As you count, notice any techniques you use to make it easier.

Question 1:

a) |||||||| ||||||||||| |||||||| ||||| |
b) |||| ||||| ||| |||| ||| |||||||| |||||||
c) |||||| ||||||| ||||||| ||||| |||| ||| |

Always be on the lookout for ways of grouping the things you're counting. Your brain is particularly open to groups of four or less, but you're likely to recognize larger groups again after you've counted them once. Sometimes several groups can be combined into new, manageable numbers – like a set of seven going with a three and being set aside in your mind as a neat group of ten.

Use the following exercise to strengthen your 'eye counting' along with your powers of visualization and memory.

Count the tally marks below. Every time you get to five marks, imagine collecting them as a group – and visualize them as a tally set of five:

Picture these sets being collected at one side of your brain. See how many sets of five you can store there comfortably, so that you can quickly say how many tally marks you've counted so far. If it helps, use your finger to keep your place on the page, but keep visualizing the growing collection of neat sets and checking how many fives you've gathered.

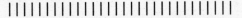

See if you can make your tallying even more efficient. This time, every time you 'collect' two sets of five, put them together as a clear group of ten, arranging the fives in pairs in your head.

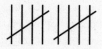

Here's the set of lines for you to tally this time:

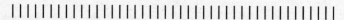

How does that feel? Does this make it even easier for you to use eyesight, imagination and mental organization to count and remember?

Unless you've grown up in a culture that deals with numbers differently, you should find it very natural to think in fives and tens. They're integral to our decimal number system – and for that we probably have our hands to thank. A natural method to help us count was at our fingertips all along.

FINGERS AND TOES

An extreme inability to calculate has been associated with damage to the part of the brain – the left parietal lobe – which controls counting on fingers, suggesting it's no coincidence that hands have played such an important part in the development of maths. We've used other things, like the counting rods popular in China for more than 2,000 years, and the knotted lengths of cords, 'quipus', favoured by the Incas of Central and South America; but fingers are the most immediate props to help us count. We even call them 'digits'. The fact that we have ten of them (or eight and two thumbs) has had a huge influence on the way we think about numbers and on the counting systems we've invented.

Of course, as well as ten fingers, we also have ten toes, so perhaps that was behind the base 20 systems developed by the Maya and Inuit cultures. A single hand's worth – base five – worked well in the Saraveca language, once spoken in Bolivia, and other South American languages formed their numbers from six to nine as five-and-one, five-and-two and so on. As long ago as the nineteenth century BCE, the Babylonians developed a number system that mixed base 60 with base ten, again showing the significance of ten in the way our counting systems have emerged, but also representing a major innovation in mathematical thinking: something called 'place value'.

The Babylonians had realized that a base set of numerals – number symbols – could be used to represent *all* the numbers they needed. The value of a particular digit depended on its position, and the spaces between them became very important. Today we use zeros in a similar way, helping to position digits and define their value, although we've refined our range of numerals to a rather simpler base of ten.

Introduced in India around 500 CE, the system we're now so familiar with was described in detail in a book published in around 825 CE by the Persian scientist Al-Khwarizmi (we'll meet him properly later in the book) but took until the twelfth century to spread to Europe. As well as a mix of Indian and Greek knowledge, it included the Arab writer's explanation of zero and its vital role in place-value thinking.

Question 2:
Exercise the memory, visualization and logic skills involved in counting by answering this question: how many times does a zero appear between 0 and 1,000?

Zero

Zero has an interesting history. The concept has been around since ancient times, meaning nothing, void; but the Ancient Greeks questioned whether 'nothing' could really be an amount at all, and went off on some typically philosophical tangents. The Olmecs of Mexico started using a symbol for zero in the fourth century BCE; and by 130 CE, the Greeks – thanks to the great mathematician Ptolemy – were using their zero symbol (a circle with a long overbar) both as a numeral in its own right, and as a placeholder to reveal important information about other digits.

Several different positional, place-value systems have been developed since ancient times. Users of counting rods and knotted ropes had learned to leave spaces, helping them to be flexible in the way they positioned their objects and to use the location of digits to determine their value, and abacus experts could display empty, 'zero' columns. But in the system we use today it's the symbol zero that plays such an important role. It can act as an amount in its own right, but it also helps to mark out the columns we visualize and to hold other digits in place.

Place value

Think about how our number system works. For example, the digit 2 represents two of something – two units – if it's written in the 'units' column, but by writing it in a different column – say, one representing thousands – that same squiggle on the page becomes a thousand times bigger. The digit 8 can become eighty, eight hundred or eight trillion, and in a vastly more efficient way than adding tally marks or simply combining numerals.

Authors' insight

If the ancient Romans had wanted to look forward to the year one thousand eight hundred and eighty eight, they would have written it as MDCCCLXXXVIII. In our present decimal place-value system, it's simply 1888.

So counting in columns was a very attractive innovation. But it was also, potentially, very confusing. In the ninth century, when the Indians had been playing with place value for 200 years and struggling with confusion about columns, they started using zeros in a revolutionary way: not just as symbols for 'nothing', but as place-holders to help structure their whole system. Their refined version of place value, based on the comfortable number 10, spread to the Middle East and then Europe by the fourteenth century and developed into the system we use in the West today. Numerals, page position and place-holding zeros combined to create a logical and efficient system that matches the decimal design of our brain.

Authors' insight

In ancient Greece, the followers of Pythagoras found magic and mysticism in numbers. They regarded the number 10 as the most holy number. It's the sum of 1, 2, 3 and 4 – which represented, respectively, existence, creation, life and the elements.

From right to left, the number 'columns' represent ones, tens, hundreds, thousands… the powers of ten, each column ten times bigger than the last. The zeros help us recognize 'empty' columns and see the exact value of each digit, and patterns of numbers emerge: 1, 10, 100, 1,000, 10,000 and so on. It's very tempting simply to add an extra 0 to make a number ten times bigger, but this only works with some types of numbers – 1.5, for example, doesn't get ten times bigger just by getting an extra zero on the end.

So it's much more useful to remember what the zero is really there for – to show that the other digits have moved to more valuable columns, increasing their worth by a factor of ten with every step. It's a good idea to strengthen your visualization skills to help you see what's going on.

To multiply 25 by ten – to make 25 ten times bigger – each digit will need to slide one space to the left, to a column 'worth' ten times more than the one where it started. To remember that the movement is left-wards, think of it as opening up more spaces for zeros to be added, showing the number getting bigger. In this case, a space comes vacant in the units column, so a zero needs to be inserted to show that the other digits have moved and to keep the columns visible.

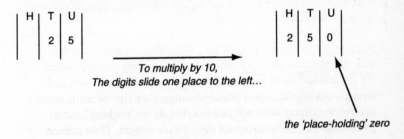

To multiply by 10,
The digits slide one place to the left...

the 'place-holding' zero

If you multiply 273 by 100, the digits will need to move two spaces to the left (the two zeros in 100 are a handy reminder), turning 273 into 27,300. Two zeros are inserted in the now empty columns, revealing the movement that's taken place.

And if the number you're working with has a decimal point, your visualization skills will help you keep it firmly in place.

To calculate 2.075 × 100, keep the decimal point where it is, slide all the digits two spaces to the left, and you'll get 207.5.

In 84.6 × 100, this sliding process opens up the units column, so just insert a zero to show that: 8,460.

And if the decimal point ends up at the far right side (for example, 36.453 × 1,000 = 36,453.) you can lose it altogether as it serves no place-value purpose.

The opposite – inverse – process to multiplication is division. To divide by powers of ten, simply do the same thing in reverse, moving all the digits to the right.

Use the following calculations to strengthen your visualization skills, your memory and your ability to follow logical instructions. Really try to 'see' the columns, keep that decimal point firmly in place, and get used to the way numbers slide left and right as you multiply or divide by powers of ten.

Question 3:

a) 47×10 b) 892×100 c) $3023 \div 100$

d) 4.38×100 e) 0.479×1000 f) $783.3206 \div 100$

g) $0.0308 \div 1000$ h) $394.30482 \times 1,000,000$

It's also good brain training to experiment with counting systems that aren't based on the number 10. It helps you to appreciate what your brain does instinctively, as well as stretching logic, visualization, memory and other key thinking skills.

Base two

Base two is binary maths. Several centuries BCE, the Indian scholar Pingala described a system in which numbers could be represented by using short or long syllables in different combinations – a bit like Morse code. Some Australian Aboriginal languages involve binary thinking. In Kala Lagaw Ya, for example, the numbers one to six look like this: *urapon, ukasar, ukasar-urapon, ukasar-ukasar, ukasar-ukasar-urapon, ukasar-ukasar-ukasar*. In the seventeenth century, German mathematician and philosopher Gottfried Leibniz invented a system using 0 and 1 which would eventually play a crucial role in the development of computers, the two digits being easily assigned to 'off' and 'on'.

In binary code, each column is twice as big as the one to the right. So, rather than units, tens, hundreds and so on, the column values look like this:

64	32	16	8	4	2	1

Working from the right, numbers are built up by inserting either 0 or 1 in each column. So 7 is written 111.

64	32	16	8	4	2	1
				1	1	1

It's like those 1s are 'switching on' the columns with the value 1, 2 and 4; and 1 + 2 + 4 = 7.

64	32	16	8	4	2	1
	1	0	0	1	1	1

The number 39 is written 100111. This time, the values switched on are 32, 4, 2 and 1, which total 39.

It's great brain training to do this mentally, converting base ten numbers to base two – and back again.

To begin, try counting up to ten in binary code. Use your mind's eye to visualize the columns, starting with 1 at the right and doubling in value to the left.

- ▶ 1 is simply 1.
- ▶ 2 is 1-0.
- ▶ 3 must be 1-1.
- ▶ 4 is 1-0-0.

Can you continue to ten?

And after that, see how far and fast can you go. It's a wonderfully logical exercise and some interesting patterns develop as the line of 1s and 0s spreads.

Authors' insight

It's been said that there are 10 types of people in the world: those who understand binary notation, and those who don't.

Question 4:

a) How quickly can you work out what 78 looks like in binary code?
b) What about 129?

Question 5:

Now try to use your brain in the other direction. Here are eight (or should that be 1000?) numbers written in binary code. Convert them to base ten in your mind. Then work out the letter value of each answer (1 = A, 2 = B, etc.) and you should discover an appropriate eight-letter word.

- ▶ 100
- ▶ 1111
- ▶ 10101
- ▶ 10
- ▶ 1100
- ▶ 1001
- ▶ 1110
- ▶ 111

THE GAME OF NIM

This is a great game for playing in the pub. It becomes very easy when you know the trick, although the maths involved provides some really powerful mental arithmetic training. Perform the key calculations smoothly and accurately and your opponent will find it almost impossible to work out what's going on – and why they always seem to lose. You, meanwhile, will have tuned up your brain power to a new level of accuracy and clarity.

Here's how to play. Three rows of coins are laid out. It's not really important how many coins there are in each row to start with (usually it depends on how many you have in your pocket) and the number of coins in each row doesn't have to be the same. The two players then take it in turns to remove any number of coins – but only from one row. The player who takes the last coin wins.

So how could you work out a strategy for a game like this?

A good start would be to simplify it. This is a typical trick of mathematicians, and a useful approach to many kinds of puzzle. If you can't solve a problem, start by considering a simpler one. Once you've got some sort of foothold, gradually make the problem harder until, with luck, you get back to the problem you wanted to solve in the first place.

So let's imagine the game has only two rows of coins.

If the rows are different lengths, the first player can guarantee a win simply by taking coins from the longer row to make the rows the same length. Then, in future moves, they mirror the move of their opponent, so that they always reduce the rows to the same length. This is a key strategy in games like this. If you make sure that you always have a move, no matter what your opponent does, then it's impossible for them to have the last move, and you have to win.

So what happens when there are three rows of coins? The key is to write the number of coins in each row not in base ten, but in base two. Why? Because in base two, each digit is either 1 or 0, representing whether a coin is still on the table or has been taken away.

Here's an example:

Coins	In base two			
	8	4	2	1
11 =	1	0	1	1
7 =	0	1	1	1
5 =	0	1	0	1
Totals	1	2	2	3

The final row shows the total number of 1s in each column. The winning strategy is this: after your move, make sure that there's an even number of 1s in each column of the base two version. This works because it's impossible for your opponent to alter these sums of 1s by more than 1, since to do so would mean removing coins from more than one row.

Your opponent can change a 2 to a 1, but never to a 0. That means you always have a move... and that means that you will certainly win the game.

So, to find the winning move for the board above, you'll need to remove an 8 and a 1. In other words, you need to take nine coins from the first row to leave:

Coins	In base two			
	8	4	2	1
2 =	0	0	1	0
7 =	0	1	1	1
5 =	0	1	0	1
Totals	0	2	2	2

At this stage your opponent has no chance. Suppose he takes six from the middle row, to leave:

Coins	In base two			
	8	4	2	1
2 =	0	0	1	0
1 =	0	0	0	1
5 =	0	1	0	1
Totals	0	1	1	2

To make the bottom totals all even, it looks like you need to remove a 4 and a 2; but there's no row with six coins. Instead, remove a 4 and add a 2, which means taking 2 coins from the last row. This gives:

Coins	In base two			
	8	4	2	1
2 =	0	0	1	0
1 =	0	0	0	1
3 =	0	0	1	1
Totals	0	0	2	2

and again all the totals are even. The noose is tightening on your opponent. Now whatever move he makes, you'll be able to reduce the game to just two rows of coins of the same length – a watertight winning position for you.

So binary notation allows your brain to try a different way of visualizing and representing numbers, warming up some key skills in the process. If you found counting from one to ten in binary code a particular stretch, it may be because of the way you normally 'see' numbers in sequence, from left to right, the direction in which we read text in the West.

Thinking about numbers

Take a moment to consider how numbers arrange themselves in your head.

Where do you 'see' zero? As numbers get bigger, do they go right-wards or upwards – or another direction altogether? Are they evenly spaced? Are all the numbers marked in your mind? Which ones are given particular prominence?

Any kind of visual model for numbers can only help you to use them. School children practise with number lines and squares, and it makes sense to strengthen whatever visual structure works for you.

Think about the way you view positive and negative numbers. Is minus 7 to the left of 0, underneath it, or somewhere else in your mind? If you calculate 16 minus 24, what are you seeing and doing in your brain?

Names in numbers: A. C. Aitken

New Zealand-born maths professor A. C. Aitken was a phenomenal mental mathematician who spent time analysing his own skills and those of other superstar thinkers. He highlighted the importance of using the things he knew about maths, especially factors and primes, and built up a rich collection of number facts. He emphasized the role of memory in his maths success and relied heavily on patterns and rhythms to structure his thinking, making the most of his advanced musical skills. Aitken wrote about some calculators who needed to talk as they worked through problems, and others who could simply visualize the concepts involved. He himself could combine both approaches: what he called a 'compound faculty'. He felt that his subconscious mind was a key part of his success. Sometimes, he said, he had the answer even before he'd decided to attempt the question.

Have a go at the following sets of instructions, keeping a running score in your memory and using whatever visual model works for you. You might imagine moving up and down a thermometer scale; or perhaps it helps to see yourself travelling in the lift of a tower block in which the ground floor is 0 and you can go down through the basement levels (-1, -2, etc.) as well as up to all the positively numbered floors.

Question 6:

a) Start at 8. Subtract 7. Add 5. Take away 10. Increase by 3. Subtract 4. Add 7.

b) $27 - 6 + 3 - 14 - 11 + 1$

c) $45 - 56 - 9 + 23 - 17 - 18 + 33$

d) $8 - 9 + 6 - 11 + 13 - 12 + 13 - 19 + 12$

And why might those four answers be significant?

An exercise like this should also reveal some key aspects of mental calculation. When the answer doesn't come instantly, most people use two core strategies when adding and subtracting in their head – based on some of the big themes of this chapter.

Partitioning involves splitting up the values of each digit (so 29 is 20 and 9; 436 is 400, 30 and 6), making the most of your inbuilt sense of place value. It requires a logical approach and good memory skills, spotting familiar combinations of numbers and keeping track of the separate bits of each calculation.

To work out 48 + 27 in this way, you'd probably think: 48 plus 20 is 68, and 68 plus 7 is 75. Or maybe, 40 plus 20 is 60, 8 and 7 are 15, 60 and 15 comes to 75.

For 84 − 27, rather than counting backwards 27 places on your mental number line, you'd probably partition 27 into 20 and 7; start by doing 84 − 20, which is 64; and then 64 − 7: 57.

Bridging uses certain numbers – usually those comfortable 10s again – as useful 'stopping points' within a calculation. You add or subtract as much as you need to get to a multiple of 10, then do whatever's left from there. Partitioning also comes in handy along the way.

So for 53 − 46 you might take away 40 from 53 to give 13, then subtract 3 to get you to the 'bridge' of 10. Finally you'd have the remaining 3 to take off: 7.

For 189 + 24 you could add 11 first to get you to 200, then add the remaining 13 from there: 213.

Both partitioning and bridging tie in closely to the way most of us were taught to calculate on paper. We might use other tactics occasionally, like rounding £2.99 to £3 and taking a penny off again later; using halving and doubling to get to an answer faster; or making the most of familiar facts about numbers. But there's much more we can do to develop a truly flexible approach. Too many people restrict themselves to a few tried-and-tested calculation strategies, whether working on paper or in their head, and don't pay enough attention to the particular numbers they're using or get to the heart of the problem in front of them. They miss out on some great opportunities to boost a whole range of thinking skills.

It's good to have a logical approach that fits the agreed system, and to match your strategies to the way your own maths mind has become structured. But you can learn to access your memory more, to spot patterns, use a few tricks here and there, and be really creative with the way you play around with numbers to make them work for you.

This chapter has explored how our mathematical system was developed and why our brains tend to handle numbers the way they do. What you can do now is start to work within that system to develop a truly flexible approach to maths and all its applications. When you do that, you extend your thinking in new directions and start reaping the benefits in many areas of your life. It's what number training your brain is all about.

NUMBER TRAINING CHALLENGES

1 Written as a word, which number has the correct number of letters?

2 If A = 1, B = 2 and so on, what is the total value of the word MATHEMATICS?

3 A desk calendar was invented that was made from two cubes. Each cube had only one digit printed on each face. Placed side by side, the cubes could be used to represent any day of the month, from 1 to 31. What was the inventor's innovative idea, and how were the digits spread between the cubes?

4 Without touching the page or writing anything down, count the letters in the full name for Bangkok:

Krung Thep Mahanakhon Amon Rattanakosin Mahinthara Yuthaya Mahadilok Phop Noppharat Ratchathani Burirom Udomratchaniwet Mahasathan Amon Phiman Awatan Sathit Sakkathattiya Witsanukam Prasit

5 What's the next number in this sequence?

11   101   111   1001

6 You've tried binary thinking, but what about *ternary*: base three. Think carefully about how it would work: just three numerals to choose from; each column three times bigger than the last...

How would someone count to ten in ternary code?

7 In a game of Nim, do you want to play first or second with the following starting positions? And if you play first, what will your move be?

a) 5, 7, 9
b) 7, 11, 13
c) 6, 9, 15

8 Use any calculating tactics you like to work through the following instructions in the order they're given. When you've found the four answers, can you spot the pattern? And what would the next number be?

a) Start at 37. Add 18. Subtract 26. Add 12. Subtract 36.
b) 100 − 72 + 44 − 80 + 39 − 23
c) Begin with 128. Divide by 2. Increase by 45. Subtract 29. Divide by 5. Decrease by 44. Add 41.
d) Multiply 378.4 by 10. Subtract 3,600. Add 128. Divide by 2. Subtract 135.

9 If someone was born in 23 BCE and died in 49 CE, what age did they live to?

10 The teacher said she was thinking of two consecutive numbers between one and ten. She told Amy one of the numbers, and Ben the other. Then the two children had the following conversation:

Amy: 'I don't know your number.'
Ben: 'I don't know yours either.'
Amy: 'I know now!'

Can you use your knowledge of numbers, your logic, memory – and any other thinking skill that helps – to work out the four possible answers to this challenge?

2

Adding skill, subtracting stress

In this chapter you will learn:
- *how addition and subtraction have been built into your brain*
- *why it's good to make the most of mathematical laws*
- *new ways to use your mind – and body – to improve your number skills*
- *brain-boosting maths puzzles and tricks.*

If I've got three apples in one hand and five apples in the other hand, what have I got? Yes, *really big hands...*

Adding makes things bigger. We know that from a very early age. An experiment with five-month-old babies and a set of Mickey Mouse toys showed that our brains *expect* 1 + 1 to be 2. When a trick was pulled on the babies, and the Mickey dolls seemed to show that 1 + 1 was 3, or 1, they were surprised, because there was already something very powerful telling them what the sum should be. Children from 18 months to three years old were shown to make very quick judgements about addition in a ping-pong ball-grabbing test. A chimpanzee was taught the number symbols and then taught himself to add two digits together.

Right from the start, the world provides us with clear pictures and meaningful experiences of what adding means. It seems our brains are set up to do it naturally. The opposite operation, subtracting, making things smaller, also comes easily. Even when we learn about negative numbers, and discover that adding can sometimes make a number smaller, the logic of increasing the debt or adding 'in the other direction' is just a natural extension of what we know.

So, whatever we go on to do with these two partner processes, addition and subtraction, we need to apply our thinking to real things whenever possible, and to make the most of the visual models we've been developing all our lives.

Starting with 'stuff'

In school, addition and subtraction are supported first by cubes, beads and other physical objects (including fingers), then by more abstract props like number lines and squares. Children learn to think of adding as going one way, taking them off on a logical journey to the right as a number gets bigger, and subtracting as moving left, decreasing the number – even beyond zero into the world of negatives and minuses.

Alongside these powerful images, key calculation strategies are established early on.

You add 1 or 2 first by 'counting on'; and, quickly, just by *knowing* the answer, your brain clicking on in sequence automatically: $3 + 1 = 4$. Subtracting by 1 or 2 is just a quick step back along the sequence.

Questions about real things quickly establish that adding or subtracting zero leaves a number unchanged, and it becomes instinctive to ignore it: $7 + 0 = 7$.

Doubling plays a role in addition from early on. We can visualize two matched amounts, understand what 'twice as much' means from simple experience, and use doubling to help us calculate quickly: $3 + 3$ (two lots of 3) $= 6$. Likewise, halving helps with subtraction, especially as the addition 'pairs' become familiar: $6 - 3 = 3$. We learn to spot and use 'near doubles' and 'near halves', for example $6 + 7$ and $14 - 8$.

As always, multiples of 5 and 10 feel easy and we can use them to simplify calculations: for example, solving $6 + 9$ by knowing that $6 + 10 = 16$ and then just subtracting 1.

Laws to live by

The **commutative** law, that $9 + 1$ is the same as $1 + 9$, is a very important concept to grasp early on, in addition at least. Children learn quickly that it's much more efficient to count up one from nine than to do it the other way round. They soon see that subtraction doesn't work in quite the same way, although the commutative principle does help to set up their brain to handle negative numbers.

Addition is also **associative,** which means that any number of addition calculations can be done in any order. It makes sense to spot ways of reorganizing a question to put certain numbers together: for example, spotting pairs of numbers that make multiples of ten. Solving 8 + 34 + 122 + 6 becomes easier simply by changing the order to 122 + 8 + 34 + 6. That is, 122 + 8 = 130, 34 + 6 = 40, and those two multiples of 10 are easily added to make 170.

Pairs of numbers are important in many calculating strategies. To be a confident mathematician you need to know all the 'number bonds' to ten (1 + 9, 2 + 8, etc.), and develop the ability to spot or calculate pairs of numbers that make 100 or 1,000. Number bonds to ten will always help. You know that 23 and 182738427 must end in zero because the last digits, 3 and 7, are bonds to ten. And you can simplify questions like 46 + 28 by adding 30 instead, then subtracting 2, because you know that the sum of numbers ending in 8 and 2 will always give you a multiple of 10.

Question 1: See how quickly you can spot the pairs of numbers that make 10.

$$4 \quad -5 \quad 1 \quad 8 \quad 14 \quad 10$$
$$0 \quad 2 \quad \quad -4 \quad 9 \quad 6 \quad 15$$

Question 2: What about larger numbers? How many number bonds to 100 can you spot here?

$$27 \quad 18 \quad 45 \quad 39 \quad 75 \quad 21 \quad \quad 73 \quad 72$$
$$41 \quad 59 \quad \quad 25 \quad 79 \quad 28 \quad 33$$

> **Authors' insight**
>
> People with particularly strong visual images for addition and subtraction are able to do complex calculations by *seeing* the answers. Skilled abacus users, for example, have been shown to use the image systems of their brains rather than typical processes of language: 'seventeen plus nine is seventeen plus ten, take away one…' Instead they have powerful visual models for what numbers look like and can quickly see the results of adding or subtracting different amounts, without having to calculate like the rest of us.

Abacus experts also understand the 'carrying' and 'borrowing' that goes on when they start dealing with larger numbers. They can visualize what's happening when they add 26 to 89 or take

75 from 164 and can see the numbers shifting between place value columns to allow each interim calculation to take place. They strengthen their memory, their ability to think logically and creatively, and their understanding of what numbers actually represent in real-life questions – so it's good for all of us to refresh some of the counting imagery we developed long ago.

It's time to flex your fingers again and boost your 'extended mind', using everything at your disposal to structure and strengthen your thinking skills.

Chisanbop

Chisanbop (from the Korean words for 'finger' and 'calculation') is a finger-counting technique that works a bit like a portable abacus. It can add a new dimension to your mental maths, but it's an absorbing brain-training challenge in its own right.

Chisanbop seems to have been developed in Korea in the 1940s, then brought to the West in the 1970s. When you know the system, you can display all the numbers from 0 to 99 on your fingers and start to explore them in a rich new way.

Hold both hands in a relaxed posture just above a table with all your fingers floating off the surface. When you start touching them against the table, you'll be indicating different values, adding and subtracting, and using Chisanbop to develop your 'digital brain'.

On your right hand, each of the four fingers has the value of one. So pressing down with the tip of your right index finger represents one. The index and the middle finger together make two, and so on.

Your right thumb is worth five when you touch it to the table on its own, but you can increase that by combining it with the other fingers. So six is made by the right thumb and index finger together, seven by the thumb and first two fingers… and onwards up to nine.

Try it for yourself. On your fingers, count up from one to nine, then back down to one. When you're comfortable with that, see how quickly you can form the following numbers on your right hand:

7   3   9   4   2   5   1   6   8

You use your left hand to represent the tens. The index finger is 10, the one next to it 20, and so on, the thumb this time representing 50 to let you count in tens all the way up to 90.

And when you start using both hands together, you can form any number from one to 99.

Show these numbers on your hands a quickly as you can:

16   28   43   83   79   3   35   55   67   99

Now have a go at adding and subtracting the Chisanbop way. As well as being a brain-stretching challenge in itself, it will exercise your logical thinking – and perhaps give you new insights into the key calculation strategies. There are certainly lessons to be learned from this task that you can apply to all the adding and subtracting you do, when shopping, doing DIY, playing Monopoly and so on.

Some numbers are quick and easy to add or subtract.

- ▶ 1 + 2: Simply show 1 on your right hand (first finger touching the table) then press down the next two fingers, to give 3.
- ▶ 9 − 3: Make 9 by using the thumb (5) and all four fingers. Then tuck in the last three fingers, revealing the answer 6: a thumb and a finger.

You quickly get the hang of using your thumbs.

- ▶ 62 + 24: Make 60 on the left hand (thumb and first finger) and 2 on the right hand (first two fingers). 24 is 20 (or 'two tens') and 4, so first add on two lots of 10 by pressing down the next two fingers on your left hand. Then you'll see that you can't simply extend four more fingers on the right, so all you do is use the thumb for 5, and tuck in a finger, since 5 − 1 is 4. You started with 62, added two 10s and 5 and subtracted 1, and now you have the answer at your fingertips: 86.

▶ 4 + 12: Begin by using your four right-hand fingers. 12 is 10 and 2, and it's easy to add the 10 with a finger on your left hand – but then you need to move on two more on your right, which involves extending the thumb and tucking in all the fingers (going from 4 to 5) and then extending the index finger to add the final one and show 6 on that hand.

The fun really starts when you need to borrow and carry.

The trick is to use complements: pairs of numbers that make 10, and multiples of 10.

▶ To calculate 3 + 9, display the 3 as usual on your right hand, but since there's no space for nine extra fingers… just add 10 (on your left hand) and subtract 1, giving 12.
▶ 46 + 38: Display 46, add on the three tens in 30, then think of the 8 as 10 − 2 as you add a 10 with one finger on the left and count back two steps on the right. (Very quickly you'll be doing this as 'add 40 and subtract 2'.)
▶ To work out 46 − 18, take away the obvious 10; then, for the remaining 8, remove another 10 and add 2 − or simply add 20 and take away 2.

Remember, when either of your thumbs is in use, subtracting 1 (one ten or one unit) will involve tucking in the thumb but extending all the fingers. You'll see what we mean when you try 55 + 39 or 62 − 34.

Try displaying and solving the following calculations as quickly as you can using this finger-waggling technique.

7 + 3   24 + 16   35 − 16   46 + 27

Now challenge yourself to answer some questions simply by looking at your hands in front of you – and resisting the temptation to move any of your digits. Can you *imagine* moving them, following the logical process you've learned until you see the final arrangement of fingers and thumbs in your mind's eye?

21 + 7   39 − 17   45 + 26   82 − 38

Question 3: Finally, try the following questions without using your hands at all. See if the 'complements' strategy can become a useful weapon in your mental maths armoury.

a) 28 + 37   b) 126 − 39   c) 303 + 269   d) 634 − 268

Thinking backwards

Number lines, abacuses, Chisanbop fingers – they all make it clear that addition and subtraction are opposite, 'inverse' operations, and help you to spot ways of using them flexibly.

See how quickly you can use subtraction to check these addition answers. Simply say whether the adding is 'right' or 'wrong' by doing a quick bit of taking away... For example:

37 + 16 = 58

> *Check: 58 − 16 = 42, not 37... so this solution is* wrong.

28 + 84 = 112

> *Check: 112 − 84 = 28... so this one is* right.

Question 4:

a) 99 + 39 = 137   b) 79 + 106 = 211   c) 239 + 425 = 664

And for the following subtraction questions, practise using addition to speed up your calculating.

For example: 35 − 19

Think: what do you have to add to 19 to make 35? 16.

Question 5:

a) 87 − 49   b) What's the difference between 74 and 39?
c) 35 − ? = 18

GET REAL

You first learned to add and subtract by thinking in real terms, using physical objects and familiar props – so it makes good sense now to relate numbers to real things whenever possible. You'll avoid making major mistakes if you continually think what the amounts you're dealing with should look like: at the start, and then as other numbers are added or taken away. You'll also switch on your visualization skills to help with logical calculations and creative solutions.

So when your seven year old says: 'If there are ten toys in a box and you take away six toys, how many have you got?' you'll be able to see the answer straight away. Yes, you've got six toys!

Question 6: There were 28 birds sitting on a fence. The farmer shot one of them. How many birds were still sitting on the fence?

Magic squares

A great way to exercise your addition strategies, along with visualization and logic, is to explore magic squares.

According to Chinese myth, back in the third millennium BCE, Emperor Yu came across a sacred turtle in a tributary of the Yellow River. The numbers 1 to 9 marked on its shell formed a remarkable pattern, because the sum of every row, column and diagonal was the same: 15.

4	9	2
3	5	7
8	1	6

In 1514, artist Albrecht Durer engraved this larger magic square – which is particularly brilliant, since the date appears at the bottom. This time the numbers one to 16 are used, and the 'magic constant' is 34.

16	3	2	13
5	10	11	8
9	6	7	12
4	15	14	1

Question 7: Can you fill in the missing numbers to finish off the following magic square? See if you can do it using your mental maths skills alone, stretching your logic to work out which numbers can and cannot appear in certain places, and putting your memory to the test as you keep track of which digits you've tried where. It's a famous example from tenth-century India and uses all the numbers from one to 16.

7		1	14
		8	
16	3	10	
	6	15	4

There are several other remarkable characteristics of this magic square. Can you spot them?

'Look ahead, borrow'

This system for subtraction also helps to strengthen your concentration and memory. As well as being a powerful brain-training tool, it can be a useful tactic for working with large numbers – especially if all you need to do is say the answer out loud.

Unlike many written methods, this system works from left to right. To demonstrate how, take the example 3,056 − 1,747.

$$3056$$
$$-1747$$

Start with the left column, the thousands. $3 - 1 = 2$; but look to the right, notice that 056 is less than 747, and 'borrow' from the thousands – which will be very helpful in a moment. So, instead of 2, say 'one'.

In the next column, the hundreds, $0 - 7$ can now be treated as $10 - 7$, which is 3; but, once again, look ahead to the right and see that 56 is greater than 47, so this time there's no need to borrow, and you can just say 'three'.

In the tens column, $5 - 4$ is 1. Look ahead and you'll see that 6 is less than 7, so you need to borrow again, and say 'zero'.

And finally in the units column, $6 - 7$ would give a negative number, but your borrowing allows you to make this $16 - 7$, giving 'nine'.

The digits you've said reveal the answer to this potentially tricky subtraction: 1309.

Question 8: Use this clever thinking system to solve the following subtractions in your head.

a) $732 - 278$ b) $3,789 - 2,815$ c) $7,832 - 5,687$

As well as logic and memory, your creativity is stretched as you look for the best ways to solve calculation puzzles.

Question 9: How quickly can you spot the key addition or subtraction strategies in the following questions?

a) $2 + \ldots\ldots = 23$ b) $\ldots\ldots + 5 = 104$
c) $45 - \ldots\ldots = 6$ d) $\ldots\ldots - 17 = 18$

Authors' insight
Don't be confused by the equals sign. Children often see it as an instruction to 'produce an answer', rather than understanding its true meaning: basically, 'is the same as'. You could use the image of weighing scales, with the equals sign in the middle, balancing equal amounts on either side.

Keypad calculations

Here's another quick exercise to practise your mental maths, boost your visualization skills and explore some intriguing patterns in numbers and shapes – all using the keypad of your mobile phone.

Start by studying your phone. Almost every phone keypad in the world arranges its number keys, 1 to 9, in the same basic way.

1	2	3
4	5	6
7	8	9

The o button will probably be underneath the 8, but you don't need to worry about that in the following activity.

After spending a few moments looking at your real keypad, practise seeing it in your mind's eye. You might imagine running your finger along each row, then each column. Use the 5 in the centre to help orientate the numbers in your mind. You could even imagine a huge keypad, big enough for you to stand on each key. Practise moving from number to number, establishing the pattern of the nine keys in your imagination.

Now test the clarity and stability of your mental keypad by completing the following calculations in your head.

▶ First, add together the digits in the four corners of the keypad and remember the total. When you've done that, spend a moment thinking about your strategy for adding these numbers. Did your brain do anything to make the calculation easier?
▶ Next, focus on the square of numbers made up by the digits in the middle of the top and bottom rows and the left and right columns. Add these four digits, remember the total – and, again, consider what you did to cope with the calculation.

If you carried out these two tasks correctly, you should have noticed the first interesting fact about the numbers on a telephone keypad.

But there's more. Try four more calculations; once again, focusing on your visualized grid of nine digits. You're strengthening your brain's ability to 'see' numbers, training yourself to process and manipulate them, and developing your awareness of significant patterns, such an important aspect of problem-solving in general.

▶ There are four lines on the grid (horizontal, vertical and two diagonals) that have the number 5 in the middle. In your mind's eye, pick out each of these lines in turn and add up each set of three digits to give you four totals.

Another fascinating fact about your mobile phone keypad should have quickly become apparent.

Do you have any theories about why this is the case? What's the link between the two activities above? See if there are any other patterns you can find as you practise visualizing and manipulating this familiar number grid.

Exercise your addition and subtraction skills the next time you do the weekly shopping. Start by estimating how much you think you'll spend; then, as you walk round the shop, keep a running total of the bill in your mind. You can either round each price to the nearest 50 pence, or stretch your memory, concentration and 'focus on the facts' even further by being accurate to the nearest penny.

Analyse all the deals on offer, subtracting any savings as you make them. Keep remembering your original estimate and checking your budget. You may well find that you change some of your purchasing habits when you start paying closer attention to prices and to the different options. You'll certainly be testing out your addition and subtraction strategies in pressurized, distracting circumstances, pushing yourself to find quick and clever ways of calculating on the move and reinforcing the connection between numbers and the real things they represent.

The 1089 trick

Here's an impressive party trick that's also a great way to practise your subtraction strategies.

Ask a friend to pick three different digits to form a three-digit number. In your head, make a second number by reversing the three digits, then subtract the smaller number from the larger one. ('Look ahead, borrow' might be the best method, but do whatever feels most comfortable for you). Next, take your answer, reverse it, and add those two numbers together. And the grand total will be… 1089 – every time.

For example: $321 - 123 = 198. 198 + 891 = 1,089$

Authors' insight

1089 is a special number. It's a perfect square, 33×33 – which may give you a clue about how this intriguing maths trick works…

NUMBER TRAINING CHALLENGES

1 Test your creativity with the following equation – which doesn't look right.

$$101 - 102 = 1$$

Can you *move* one symbol to make it correct?

2 Think flexibly about the following numbers to find five pairs with the sum of 26.

$$-4 \quad 12 \quad 13$$
$$15 \quad 2 \quad -5 \quad 10 \quad 18$$
$$13 \quad -6 \quad 14 \quad 30 \quad 24 \quad 32$$

3 Picture the digits 1 to 9 in sequence. It's possible to place + and – symbols in this line to bring the total to 100. For example:
$$1 + 2 + 34 - 5 + 67 - 8 + 9 = 100$$

There are at least 11 other ways to do it. How many of them can you find?

4 In the Fibonacci sequence, every number is the sum of the previous two. After 0, the sequence starts: 1, 1, 2, 3, 5, 8… Challenge yourself to continue this logical sequence in your mind. See if you can find the first 20 numbers.

5 Remind yourself of the Chisanbop finger-counting technique (see earlier in this chapter), then use it to answer the following questions as quickly as you can. And if you're in the mood for a challenge, try doing it entirely in your imagination.

a) $25 + 37$ b) $304 - 25$ c) $173 + 258$ d) $236 - 167$

6 Find the cleverest ways to solve the following addition questions in your head.

a) $89 + 88$ b) $123 + 288$ c) $384 + 7,236$
d) $1,902 + 30,401$

7 Using only the numbers 1 to 16, can you complete the magic square below? The magic constant is 34.

	6	3	
4			5
	1	8	
7			2

8 Use your strengthened subtraction skills to solve the following questions as quickly as possible.

a) 23 − 14   b) 345 − 250   c) 437 − 358
d) 3,748 − 1,809

9 For the next set of questions, challenge yourself to use the 'Look ahead, borrow' technique (explained earlier in this chapter).

a) 65 − 47   b) 248 − 178   c) 374 − 285
d) 2,374 − 1,387

10 Test your memory, concentration and flexible approach to calculating by following these addition/subtraction instructions. Carry out the steps in order, then use the system A = 1, B = 2, etc. to turn your four answers into letters that can be rearranged into an appropriate word.

a) 235 − 26 + 49 − 253
b) 809 + 374 + 234 − 789 − 608
c) 38 + 39 − 104 + 28 − 328 + 400 − 53
d) 1000 − 222 − 333 + 404 + 515 − 1,234 + 4,321 − 4,432

3

Multiply your mind power:
divide and conquer

In this chapter you will learn:
- *creative approaches to multiplication and division*
- *why visualization is vital to good mathematical thinking*
- *tips for mastering times tables*
- *calculating techniques that will help you train your brain for anything.*

Our maths minds may be built on foundations of addition and subtraction, but very soon we're faced with two new challenging ideas: multiplication and division. And, for many of us, this is where the problems start. Our understanding of what numbers can do is stretched in new ways: not just backwards and forwards along the line of numbers running through our heads, but off and out into the daunting space opened up by multiplication – and then back again, as division starts to do some truly brain-bending things...

Authors' insight

Maybe the ancient Babylonians and Egyptians had it right. They employed scholars to construct huge times-table charts, so that the rest of them could avoid the task of multiplying altogether.

Computers don't really do multiplication or division either. Instead they do high-speed addition and subtraction; and the good news is that many of the techniques explored in the last chapter will come in handy again here. As you train your maths brain, you learn to use all four operations ($+ - \times \div$) flexibly, finding clever ways to pick and choose the right tools for the job. All the key thinking skills you've been exercising will also come into their own as you tackle some challenging concepts and experiment with further ways to use your brain at its best. As the title of this chapter suggests, there's a great deal to be gained from mastering multiplication and dominating division. You'll gain key maths skills to help you with a range of real-life challenges, but you'll also continue the valuable process of training your brain to cope with anything.

As with addition and subtraction, it's very useful to understand that multiplication and division are inverse operations. In school, these processes are introduced as new ways of making things bigger or smaller, and that's certainly where we need to start – even if those comfortable concepts are soon called into question. Multiplication and division will prove to be rather more complicated ($2 \times \frac{1}{2}$, $3 \div 0.6...$), although the idea of them being opposite operations, 'building up' or 'breaking down' numbers in stages, is still a very useful analysis of what's going on.

Question: What multiplies by division?

Answer: An amoeba.

The vocabulary itself starts to multiply at this point. Now we have 'times', 'lots of', 'product', 'multiple', 'factor', 'share'… and it becomes particularly important to be logical and focused in the way the language of maths is used. Miss key details and you can easily go wrong.

What do you get when you divide 16 by a half?

The typical reply to this question is 8, but the right answer is 32. Dividing by a half is very different from 'cutting in half' – dividing by 2 – which is what the question *sounds* like it wants you to do.

On the other hand, phrase a question in a slightly different way and you give yourself a much better chance of cracking it.

Calculate $\frac{1}{2} \times 24$.

Most people have no problem with this question if it's rephrased slightly: 'calculate $\frac{1}{2}$ *of* 24'.

Leaps of faith

If you think carefully about what a multiplication or division question involves, your personal mental arrangement of numbers – your own 'number line' – can continue to be of great help. Children might be shown how to visualize the 3 times table by seeing all the 'jumps' of 3 along the number line: from 0 to 3, then to 6, 9, 12... Wherever this journey stops, they can look back at all the three-size steps that got them there, dividing their final number into clearly equal chunks.

For a question like 4×45, the number line lets you fix on 45 to start with, think about its value in terms of the distance from 0, then build up in three more equal steps of 45: to 90, 135 and finally 180. You can see how the multiplication answer was achieved and what 4×45 looks like – and the link with division is clear: that 180 can be divided, broken down again, into those four number-line sections of 45.

Arrays

Another visualization tactic is to think about arrays – for example, four rows of five dots, apples, abacus beads or anything else is what 4×5 'looks like'. It provides you with clear, visual proof of the 'commutativity' of multiplication – that, like addition, it doesn't matter which way round you do it: 2×3 is the same as 3×2. An array of ten rows by two rows can become an array of two-by-ten simply by looking at it in a slightly different way.

It also confirms the connection between multiplication and division. A ten-by-five array of golfballs in a box shows $10 \times 5 = 50$, but also reveals that those 50 balls can be divided into five rows of ten, or ten rows of five. It demonstrates that division can be about dividing into particular-sized groups, or sharing between a certain number. Suddenly a whole set of useful facts emerges from the one place, prompting you to use these two operations in harmony as you strengthen and flex your maths brain.

If you know that 2×3 is 6, 3×2 must be 6 too; but you can also say that $6 \div 3$ is 2, and $6 \div 2$ is 3. You're much more likely to see that $30 \div 7.5 = 4$ if you realize you already know that $4 \times 7.5 = 30$.

In the following questions, use multiplication to check division facts, and vice versa. Practise manipulating the numbers in your head to say quickly whether each of these equations is *right* or *wrong*.

Question 1:

a) $69 \div 3 = 23$ b) $81 \div 27 = 4$ c) $38 \div 19 = 2$
d) $6 \times 25 = 155$ e) $36 \times 4 = 144$ f) $30 \times 12 = 366$

Building this sort of understanding into your brain sets it up for efficient calculation, increasing your store of useful number facts and giving you some very accurate ways of checking your ideas. It helps you to estimate well, lets you spot connections between numbers, and prepares your brain to choose sensible calculating strategies. You're thinking carefully about the values and shapes of numbers, not just the digits that represent them on the page.

Abacus users know the power of thinking in arrays. They might spot that an array of 2×7 beads contains within it 2×5, a clear and manageable set of 10, plus 2×2 more. An array of 10×4 oranges could be seen as 5 rows of 8: so $40 \div 8$ is 5, and $40 \div 5$ is 8. Experiments have shown that abacus experts develop very clear mental models like this so that, before long, the only abacus they need is in their head. Brain scans show them thinking in pictures: quickly, accurately and creatively.

So when you come to multiply or divide on paper, you should be ready to deal with the whole problem in front of you: the full value of the numbers involved and the full extent of the things that need to be done to them.

Written rules

The 'grid method' of multiplication, and the 'chunking' style of division, now popular in schools, represent a move towards written methods that are based on understanding the true value of numbers, not just dealing with the digits on the page. As with addition and subtraction, they rely on a strong sense of place value and the ability to partition numbers. They work logically, but there's also room for creativity and a few clever mental moves.

In the grid method, you show very clearly how every part of the first number needs to be multiplied by every part of the second. Addition skills are also brought in to help.

You choose to partition numbers as much as you need, arrange them in a grid pattern, then carry out all the individual multiplications – before adding the answers to produce the grand total.

Your grid for 306 × 498 would probably look like this:

×	400	90	8
300			
6			

Then you'd fill in the answers, using any mental multiplication strategy that helped.

×	400	90	8
300	1200	27000	2400
6	2400	540	48

Your addition sum would then be:

$$
\begin{array}{r}
1200 \\
27000 \\
2400 \\
2400 \\
540 \\
+ 48 \\
\hline
33588 \\
11
\end{array}
$$

In the chunking method of division, subtraction provides the key to breaking down a number as much as you possibly can. You think about the value of the figures in front of you, then see how many times you can subtract one number from the other.

A typical way of recording it all on paper looks like this:

$$24\overline{)549}$$

The question is: how many times can you take 24 out of 549?

Or...

▶ if we divided 549 into 24 groups, how many would be in each group?
▶ if we wanted to make groups of 24 out of 549, how many groups would there be?
▶ what number is 24 times smaller than 549?

You could start by subtracting 10 lots of 24, 240, making a note of what you'd done and calculating the new, reduced amount.

```
  2 4 | 5 4 9
      |
    – 2 4 0 | × 10
      3 0 9 |
```

Then you'd see that you could do the same thing again and take out another 10 lots of 24:

```
  2 4 | 5 4 9
      |
    – 2 4 0 | × 10
      3 0 9
    – 2 4 0 | × 10
        6 9
```

So, after taking 24 out of 549, 20 times, you'd be down to 69. You could then subtract it twice more...

```
  2 4 | 5 4 9
      |
    – 2 4 0 | × 10
      3 0 9
    – 2 4 0 | × 10
        6 9
        4 8 | × 2
        2 1
```

... after which you'd have to stop, after taking it out 22 times, with 21 spare. So 549 divided by 24 is '22 remainder 21'. It looks rather different on a calculator, and we'll explore remainders as we delve further into divided numbers in the next chapter; but the beauty of this system is that you can follow the whole process very clearly, and use a range of calculating strategies along the way to the final answer.

It's good practice for your logical processing, visualizing and remembering to try both of these techniques mentally.

Without writing anything down, see if you can use a grid method arrangement in your mind to solve the following multiplications. Take the opportunity to think about the maths strategies and thinking skills you use along the way.

Question 2:

a) 23×42 b) 71×45 c) 241×33 d) 103×420

Now have a go at chunking your way to answering some division questions. Think carefully about the most useful numbers to subtract, work hard to keep track of the 'subtraction count', and once again pay attention to your instinctive calculation strategies.

Question 3:

a) $320 \div 15$ b) $414 \div 35$ c) $520 \div 21$ d) $570 \div 45$

Both these systems are 'transparent', meaning that you can see what's going on inside, and giving them a clear advantage over many of the other written methods that have been developed.

Most of us have been taught ways of multiplying and dividing that work perfectly well, even though we don't really know *how* they work. In this chapter we'll introduce you to some new techniques as part of the brain-training process, helping you to strengthen your memory and exercise your concentration and focus. But even in these there's plenty of conscious calculating to do, continually developing key aspects of your mental maths and helping to reveal the bigger picture.

The more you can see and understand what's going on in your head, the further you can go with your mathematical thinking, the more cleverly it can be applied to a variety of other challenges, and the more useful brain training you can extract from the whole experience.

So before the challenge of new systems, let's look at the key strategies. You may well have just spotted some of them in action. There are some powerful thinking habits to get into that will make grappling with numbers as pain-free as possible, and strengthen key areas of your maths brain in the process.

Sensible strategies

Pay attention to the way in which you order your calculations. We've seen that the *commutative* law applies to multiplication. If you're paying 3p a minute for a call lasting 250 minutes, 250 × 3 is the same as 3 × 250, and '3 lots of 250' is a much easier concept for your brain to tackle than '250 lots of 3.'

Get used to thinking in manageable units: a few big things rather than many small ones.

The *associative* law is helpful, too, because you can order the steps of a multiplication to suit the way your brain works. Work through 125 × 99 × 2 × 4 in your head, in the order in which it's written, and you'll find it much harder to handle than if you'd changed it to 4 × 125 × 2 × 99. The second version pairs up numbers that are much easier to calculate, and the interim answers are memorable: 500 × 2 = 1,000; 1,000 × 99 = 99,000. Do everything you can to *make* information memorable.

Take every opportunity to use the *compensation* principle. Those multiples of 10 are always easiest to cope with: so, for 19 × 4, it makes sense to calculate 20 × 4 first and then take away 4. It's particularly important in matters of money: 3 × £8.99 is much more manageable if you treat the price as £9, multiply that by 3, then remember to subtract the three pennies you added to make the maths easier. Be flexible and creative in your mental organization.

You can also combine processes creatively. Division can help you to multiply. Multiplying by five is usually much easier to think of as multiplying by ten and then dividing by two. To multiply a number by nine, first multiply by 10 and then subtract the starting number.

As well as multiples of five and ten, other numbers are particularly useful when you're multiplying or dividing. You have much more flexibility with a number boasting plenty of *factors* – the numbers that can be multiplied to form it. For example, 12 has the whole-number factors 1, 2, 3, 4, 6 and 12, so you can divide the 12 months of the year or the 12 hours of the day in a variety of ways. To multiply something by 12 you could multiply it by six and then by two, or by three and then by four if that was easier.

History's great mental mathematicians have often used factors to help them, and we've structured key aspects of life on highly 'composite' numbers – like 360: degrees in a circle, days in the Babylonian calendar and so on.

Question 4: How quickly can you pick out all the whole-number factors of 360? There are certainly plenty of them! Give your concentration and memory a workout by listing them all – and counting just how many factors 360 has to offer.

Focusing on the key facts and using the logic of factorization can simplify things greatly. For example:

16×20 is the same as $16 \times 2 \times 10$.

If you'd calculated that 14×15 was 211, you'd be able to use factors (in this case, 7 and particularly 2 and 5) to realize you'd gone wrong: 211 clearly isn't a multiple of 2 or 5.

18×24 could be cracked by thinking of it as $18 \times 8 \times 3$, or $18 \times 2 \times 12$, or $18 \times 6 \times 4$, or $18 \times 6 \times 2 \times 2$, which is 108 doubled and doubled again: 432.

Authors' insight

A crucial theme throughout this book is taking control of numbers, visualizing, remembering, ordering, patterning and being creative with them until they fit the way *your* brain works best.

Doubling and halving

Doubling and halving are processes that feel natural and work smoothly in our brains. Creativity and logic come together powerfully as you find ways to make the most of these special operations. It's much easier to calculate 4×17 when you think of it as 'double 17 and double again'. $360 \div 4$ is simplified by halving it and then halving it again. The ancient Egyptians did a great deal of their maths with the help of doubling tables. Doubling and halving can also be used powerfully in combination, reframing questions to make them much more straightforward. For example, 26×32 is the same as 52×16, 104×8, 208×4, 416×2... so $26 \times 32 = 832$.

Put your creative, flexible maths mind to the test now with the following set of questions. Pick and choose from the many thinking strategies you've learned to boost your accuracy, increase your calculating speed, and continue your brain training.

Question 5:

a) $40 \times 87 \times 2 \times 25 \times 5$ b) 29×8 c) 190×3
d) 64×9 e) 12×80

Ordered thinking

You know that there's no difference between $6 + 7$ and $7 + 6$, and 8×9 gives the same answer as 9×8. Subtraction is the opposite of addition, and division the opposite of multiplication. But... what happens when these operations are mixed up in a single question? Does it matter which way round you do things?

This question should show that it does: what is $2 + 3 \times 4$? Most people would work from left to right: $2 + 3 = 5$, $5 \times 4 = 20$. The correct answer is actually 14: $3 \times 4 = 12$, $2 + 12 = 14$.

The agreed rule is that you always do multiplication and division first before addition and subtraction. And if you need to choose between multiplying and dividing, or whether to add or subtract, you just work from left to right.

Question 6: Hold this rule in your memory and exercise your ordered thinking as you calculate the correct answers to the following questions. And then, if you've got any mental energy left, why not see what happens when you forget the rule and just go left to right…?

a) $10 + 20 \times 30 \div 40 - 50$
b) $100 - 8 \times 3 + 12 \div 4$
c) $17 + 80 \div 2 \times (7 + 3) - 17$
d) $6^2 + (\sqrt{81} \times 2) \div 6 - 10 \times 3$

The Syracuse algorithm

This is an interesting exercise for your concentration, visualization and memory. Start with any number you want, then:

▶ if it's even, divide it by two
▶ if it's odd, multiply it by three and add one.

After that, repeat the process with your answer… and keep doing it, until you get to the cycle 4, 2, 1, 4, 2, 1. Mathematicians believe that you will always slip into this pattern – although sometimes it will take a while. Try it with 27, for example…

Question 7: As you put the number 27 through the Syracuse algorithm, can you also keep a mental note of how many steps it takes to fall into the 4, 2, 1 cycle? If you're right, the answer is an interesting number in itself!

Times tables

Among all the sound strategies for thinking about multiplication, understanding processes and patterns and making quick mental calculations, there's still a very important place in number training for instant recall of times tables. It may seem an old-fashioned aspect of maths education, but it fits in well with the modern brain-training principle of repeating simple calculations to strengthen nerve connections – making physical changes to support thinking. However old you are, it pays to perfect your times tables, boosting your speed and accuracy with many of the brain-training activities in this book – and their applications in real life.

TIMES TABLE TIPS

Focus on the facts. Think about all the facts you already know well. You shouldn't have any problem with the one times table, or the tens, since your brain has developed to cope with these patterns. Twos and fives should also come naturally, especially when you get used to switching numbers as necessary ('12 times 2' is probably as easy to cope with as 'two twelves') and using doubling and halving: remember, five times anything is the same as ten times, then halved. The pattern of the 11 times table – 11, 22, 33... – should make it all very easy to remember.

Play some tricks. When you've highlighted the facts you still need to master, think about any multiplication tricks that could help: doubling, halving, compensating... Four times anything is 'double and double again'; eight times is 'double, double, double'. To calculate 9×7, why not do 10×7 and then take away 7? Use the answers you do know to help deliver the ones you still find hard.

Maximize your memory. When you find answers that still won't come quickly, why not use a few memory strategies to imprint them on your brain?

▶ Imagine writing '$6 \times 7 = 42$', '$8 \times 9 = 72$' or whatever, in large, brightly coloured numbers. Hold them in your mind's eye as you extract some of the other facts they hold: like $42 \div 7 = 6$ or $72 \div 8 = 9$. Think about what the numbers mean, at the same time as focusing on what they look like in this bright, clear writing in your head. You might even play around with the shape of the digits and the sound of the answers.

▶ The number 8 looks a bit like a snowman; 7 could be a desk lamp. Imagine if you shone a lamp onto a snowman and it melted, leaving behind nothing but a pair of 'filthy socks' – 'fifty six'!

▶ 6 could be b, 9 looks like q: so how about using a barbeque to cook a 'fluffy paw', 54... These weird images and phrases may be just what your brain needs to hold on to the last few elusive answers.

Practise. Repeat the times tables until you're used to their rhythms, the sounds of the words, the feel of the facts in your head. Knowing these key multiplications instantly is a really important and beneficial aspect of developing a number-trained brain.

Question 8: Give your brain a quick fire workout with this set of times tables.

a) 4×7 b) 8×8 c) 3×6 d) 12×5 e) 9×6

f) 7×11 g) 4×6 h) 7×8 i) 3×9 j) 6×7

k) 5×9 l) 8×4 m) 3×12 n) 9×4 o) 8×6

DIGITAL NINES

Has anyone ever shown you the 'extended mind' technique of using your hands to sort out the nine times table?

Hold your ten digits in front of you. Think of them as representing the numbers 1 to 10, going from left to right. For any nine-times-table fact, simply put down the appropriately-numbered finger. (So, to get three nines you'd put down finger number three; for seven nines, the seventh finger from the left.)

When you've done that, think of the finger you've moved as a gap separating tens from units. So, if you've put down finger four, to get 4×9, you'll see that your hands are now showing three tens on one side of the gap and six units on the other: 36. Finger nine drops down to show that 9×9 is eight tens and one unit: 81. All the nine-times-table answers are at your fingertips!

THE GUESS-MY-AGE MACHINE

Ask a volunteer to multiply their age by ten and then to subtract any number in the nine times table up to 9×9, 81. When they tell you their final answer, simply look at the digits and do a quick bit of addition to decode their age.

If they're 30, $30 \times 10 = 300$; and if they chose to subtract 2×9, 18, their answer would be 282. 28 years plus two years tells you their age. A 72-year-old volunteer would get 720, take away say 27 to give 693. $69 + 3 = 72$.

Techniques and tricks

We promised a few new systems to challenge your number training. Have a go at the following ingenious techniques, pushing yourself to learn the instructions, follow the logic, visualize the key steps, keep a running record of any interim answers... and think about any creative uses you could put them to in real-life calculations.

46

MULTIPLYING BY 11

First, make a mental note of the 'ones' digit in the multiplier (in 43 × 11 this would be the 3) and use this to create a temporary result, which you'll be building into the full solution. Then, starting with that number, add each digit in the multiplier to the digit on its left. Every time you get an answer, add it to the left of the temporary result. If it's more than 9, carry the 1 (ten) over to the next addition. Finally, take the first number of the multiplier (adding a carried 1 if necessary) and make this the first number in the temporary result – which now just happens to be the final answer!

So, for 175 × 11, the 'ones' digit is 5	temporary result = 5
5 + 7 = 12	temporary result = 25 ('carry 1')
7 + 1 = 8 + the carried 1 = 9	temporary result = 925
The first number of the multiplier = 1	final result = 1,925

Have a go yourself. For the first couple of questions below, follow the instructions in the text and use pencil and paper if necessary. But then challenge yourself to do it all mentally, visualizing the temporary result as it grows into the permanent solution.

Question 9:

a) 24 × 11   b) 382 × 11   c) 436 × 11
d) 2,738 × 11   e) 94,938 × 11

SPEED MATHS CHALLENGE

Here's a great way to use this × 11 technique to show off your number training – and maybe even to win some money in the process.

Ask your friend to write down any two single-digit numbers, one above the other. Between you, keep adding each number to the one above it until you have a stack of ten numbers on the page. Then the challenge is to add up all ten numbers: the fastest person wins.

And, to win… all you need to do is look at the *fourth number from the bottom* and multiply it by 11. Put the system you've just learned into practice and win the bet every time.

··

Authors' insight

111111111 is an interesting number. Multiplied by itself, the answer is 12345678987654321.

··

'VERTICALLY AND CROSSWISE'

This is a multiplication system taken from Vedic maths, a system of 16 basic principles outlined by the Hindu mathematician Bharati Krishna Tirthaji Maharaja in the early twentieth century. It's particularly useful for tackling larger two-digit numbers, and puts your visualization and organized thinking to the test.

You need to picture your four numbers in the following square arrangement:

```
3              8
       ×
2              9
```

First multiply the verticals: 3×2 and 8×9, putting the answers below each one. If an answer is greater than 9, carry the tens unit into the next column along. In this example, 3×2 is fine as 6; but 8×9 is 72, so the 2 goes under the right-hand vertical and the 7 into a column in the middle:

```
3              8
       ×
2              9
_____
6      7       2
```

Then multiply the diagonals and add the two answers together, placing that total between the previous two. If there's already a carried digit in that position, just add it on, and carry anything extra into the column under the left-hand vertical. In this case, $(2 \times 8) + (3 \times 9) = 43$. There's already a 7 in place, so that makes 50. Put the 0 next to the 2 and carry across the 5, turning the 6 into 11:

```
   3              8
          ×
   2              9
_____
1     1     0      2
```

So your answer is 1,102.

Try it yourself. The first two questions are fairly straightforward as they don't involve any carrying of digits. The other two do, and are fantastic opportunities to feel the emerging power of your number-trained brain.

Question 10:

a) 12×13 b) 21×23 c) 16×37 d) 55×66

Here's another handy multiplication method. It works for any two numbers from 11 to 19 and it gives you an extra strategy to add to your mental maths repertoire, sharpening your mind's ability to visualize, organize and process information in the most efficient way.

Picture the larger of the two numbers on top of the other, for example:

1 7
1 3

Next, imagine drawing a line around the top two digits and the digit at the bottom right: in this case the 17 and the 3. Add these two numbers together, 20, then multiply the result by ten, which in practice just means putting a zero at the end: 200.

Staying within the shape you drew, multiply the digit at the bottom right by the digit above it: $3 \times 7 = 21$.

Finally, simply add these two totals together: $200 + 21 = 221$.

Try it on paper first, then practise visualizing the four digits as clearly as possible as you carry out these straightforward steps in your mind.

To help you remember the two totals for long enough to combine them:

▶ 'say' the numbers loudly and clearly in your mind
▶ imagine writing the numbers in your best handwriting
▶ see the numbers drawn with bright colours or picked out in neon lights.

Take every real-life opportunity you get to practise this and all the other techniques explored in this chapter. Multiplication and division challenges present themselves daily: working out if the multi-buy deals really are good value; splitting up the restaurant bill so that everyone's happy; calculating quantities to make the recipe feed the whole family; reading map scales to see how far you've still got to hike... Choose carefully from the key calculating strategies and try out a few of the new systems. As well as boosting your speed, improving your accuracy and increasing your confidence with numbers, you'll be sharpening your brain as you strengthen some of the most important thinking skills of all.

NUMBER TRAINING CHALLENGES

1 Can you find the cleverest ways to solve the following multiplications?

   a) 29×12 b) 16×140 c) $4 \times 16 \times 5 \times 2$ d) 198×8

2 See how quickly you can complete the following calculation, using any thinking skills that might help:

   $1 \times 2 \times 3 \times 4 \times 5 \times 6 \times 7 \times 8 \times 9 \times 0$

3 Use some of your addition techniques from Chapter 2 to help with these multiplications:

   a) $1{,}463 \times 2$ b) 845×3 c) $1{,}382 \times 4$

4 Can you set up mental grids to solve the following multiplication questions?

   a) 2×79 b) 16×17 c) 123×4 d) 210×14

5 Use the 'vertically and crosswise' strategy (see 'Techniques and tricks' in this chapter) to solve some more multiplication problems:

   a) 11×18 b) 13×14 c) 22×33

6 Use the 'chunking' method (see 'Written rules' in this chapter), mentally if you can, to solve these divisions.

   a) $135 \div 5$ b) $184 \div 8$ c) $414 \div 9$

7 Test your creativity with this halving problem. Your next-door neighbour has three children, and half of them are girls. How can that be possible?

8 Which of your thinking skills will help you to solve this famous division puzzle? You want to use an old gold chain to pay your gardener for seven days of service. The chain has seven links on it, and you've agreed that the gardener will earn one link per day. He won't work without receiving his day's pay each afternoon,

but you don't want to give him more than his daily fee in case he doesn't return. So, you'll need to cut some of the links on the chain to make the daily payments. What's the smallest number of links you need to cut so that your gardener receives only one link each day? And would it help if the worker agreed not to spend his money until the end of the week...?

9 Imagine you've been placed on a course of expensive medication and you need to take one tablet of medicine A and one tablet of medicine B every day. You have to be careful to take just one of each because there could be some serious side effects. Taking an A without a B, or vice versa, should also be avoided because these tablets need to be taken together to work. So... you open up the A bottle and tap one pill into your hand. You put that bottle aside and you open the B bottle – but, by mistake, two Bs fall into the hand holding the A pill. So now you've got a problem. The A and B pills look and feel identical. So what are you going to do? How can you make sure that you get your daily dose of exactly one A and exactly one B without wasting any of the pills?

10 A farmer had four sons and 15 sheep. He decided to give half his sheep to his first child, half of the remaining sheep to son number two, half of what was left to the third boy and then half of the remainder to his final child. How did he do it?

4

....

Bits and pieces

In this chapter you will learn:
- *strategies for coping with decimals and fractions*
- *the importance of keeping your brain in balance*
- *how to grapple with the mind-bending issue of zero*
- *why handling percentages can boost a wide range of thinking skills.*

Question 1: What can you put between five and nine to produce a number bigger than five and smaller than nine?

The last chapter revealed how multiplication and division are built into the very fabric of our mathematics. The number system we use multiplies the value of digits tenfold towards the left, for ever; and however far you've gone, you can just as easily shuffle them back to the right, dividing by ten each time through thousands, hundreds, tens and units. But of course it doesn't stop there. There's an exciting realm to the right of the units, into values less than a whole: tenths, hundredths, thousandths… again, on and on as far as you want to go. The clearest markings on our mental number line may be the whole numbers, but we also have to get used to seeing all the values in between.

A number-trained brain is focused and logical in its approach to the 'bits and pieces' of decimals, fractions, ratios and percentages, as well as being creative enough to handle some of the big ideas they open up.

As we develop our maths minds we begin with whole numbers, but very quickly we're thinking about values less than a whole: bits of cake, chapters of books, hours in the day. We learn to handle the pennies that make up pounds, the steps required to finish a task, the different ways available to describe the constituent bits. We also discover how useful it is to be able to compare amounts, to see the relative significance of individual pieces, and to use the 'numbers in between the numbers' to understand and describe a distinctly fractured world.

For thousands of years people have been struggling with division, grappling with its implications for mathematical thinking. The Romans only split amounts as much as common business practice required. Before them, the Egyptians had restricted their thinking to single bits, fractions with a 1 at the top – apart from 2/3 and 3/4 – and the Babylonians' system, with its columns of sixtieths, then three-thousand-six-hundredths, was limited by its confusing lack of anything like a decimal point. Indian mathematicians incorporated fractions into their decimal system around 500 CE, after which the system spread to Europe via the Arabic world, picking up new techniques for representing part-values clearly along the way.

Fibonacci was using fractions in the thirteenth century. In the 1500s, Simon Stevin published a method for representing fractions as decimals, labelling the columns to the right of the units to make it clear that they were very different from those on the left. It was the French who eventually started using commas to make the distinctions, while others preferred points and full stops to separate the whole numbers from the bits.

It's a challenge to explore values less than a whole, especially when you start applying them to calculations and trying to fit them into the wider number system. The areas of mathematical thinking and working we deal with in this chapter offer some powerful opportunities for brain training.

There are so many different ways of thinking about the same scenario.

Imagine this one: a group of ten children, of which four are girls and six are boys.

A girl in that group is one of ten children – 1/10 – and that fraction fits nicely with our base ten system, where we just need to put a 1 in the 'tenths' columns, the space with a value ten times smaller than the units column to the left of it: 0.1

The *set* of girls, four of them, could be described as 4/10 – or, more simply, as 2/5 – as well as 0.4. They also represent 40 per cent of the whole group, helping you to compare the proportions here with those in *any* group. For each two girls there are three boys, so we can talk in terms of ratios. Here, the ratio of girls to boys is 2:3. Divided into five parts, gender pairs, two of those parts are girls and three of them boys.

It's good to have a brain flexible enough to cope with all the different ways of expressing complex amounts.

Balance your brain

Logic helps you to understand systems and follow rules. Use the following exercises to boost your 'balanced thinking', making sure you keep both sides of each equation in proportion. See how quickly you can you convert…

Question 2: … between fractions: for example, ½ = 5/10. Remember, however much you multiply or divide the top number, you have to do exactly the same to the one on the bottom.

a) 1/4 = …/40   b) 3/5 = …/20
c) 3/20 = …/1000   d) 1 ½ = …/180

Question 3: … between fractions and decimals: e.g. ½ = 0.5. Think about the columns you're working in now: tenths, hundredths, thousandths…but also use key number facts you know.

a) 1.75 = …   b) 4/5 = …
c) 33.333… = …   d) 60/80 = …

Question 4: … between fractions, decimals and percentages: e.g. ½ = 0.5 = 50%. Just think of percentages as fractions with the bottom number of 100.

a) 2/5 = …%   b) 1.8 = …%
c) 72% = …/25   d) 122% = 1 …/…

Question 5: And now, how flexibly can you use your skills to solve the following mixed questions? When you've had a go, look back through them and think about the different calculating and thinking skills you used.

a) 0.75 = …%   b) 6/51 = …/17
c) 1/5 = 0. …   d) 48% = 12/…

Your ability to focus on the facts and to visualize key aspects of a question becomes particularly important when you're dealing with decimals and fractions. This is partly because we've built an idea into our brains about multiplication increasing and division decreasing – but that only works for whole numbers.

1 × 40 is 40 ('one of 40') ... so when anything less than 1 is used to multiply, the answer will get smaller. 0.9 × 40 is 36, 9/10 of 40.

Think carefully about this next one. What is 1/4 divided by 1/2? Remember, this isn't the same as 'divided by 2': in fact, it's the opposite. It's more like saying 'how many halves are in one quarter'. 1/4 ÷ 1/2 = 1/2 is quite a brain-stretching idea.

Question 6:

a) What is 1/2 × 1/2?   b) 0.4 ÷ 5 = ?   c) Calculate 0.75 × 72

You need to train your brain to consider the value of each amount in front of you, rather than getting confused by the individual digits (a 9 isn't always worth more than a 1) or by similar-looking amounts (0.75 and 74 are very different).

Visualization is vital. Picture the amounts in question, not the numbers, and try to apply your calculations to real things.

For example, 1/3 × 3/10 can be calculated logically by multiplying top and bottom numbers to give 3/30, then dividing both numbers by three to give 1/10. But picturing 'one third of three tenths' would probably tell you much faster that the answer is one tenth.

What about 1/2 divided by 1/4? The rule says turn the second fraction upside down and then multiply horizontally: 1/2 × 4/1. But it's much more useful to you if you're in the habit of picturing half a cake and just 'looking' to see how many quarter cakes it contains: clearly, 2.

With fractions, logic only takes you so far. You need to be prepared to cope with the unpredictability of division. Multiply whole numbers and you'll get more whole numbers, always; but divide and the results are uncertain.

Question: Is there a way you can divide seven identical pieces of bread equally among 12 people?

Answer: You cut three of the pieces of bread in four and the other four pieces of bread in three. So you have 12 thirds and 12 quarters. Now everyone can take a third and a quarter and receive an equal amount of bread.

Building up an 'instinct for divisibility' taps your brain into some fundamental aspects of mathematical thinking. In division problems, it's often very useful to know whether a number or amount is divisible neatly by another. It helps when you're measuring up for DIY jobs, ordering party food or sorting teams on the training ground. It also offers some good number-training exercise.

Divisibility tricks

A number is only divisible by three if the sum of its digits is too. So 283,746 must be divisible by three because $2 + 8 + 3 + 7 + 4 + 6 = 30$, and 30 certainly is!

More of a challenge for your memory skills is the trick for checking divisibility by seven.

- ▶ Step 1: Remove and double the last digit of the number in question.
- ▶ Step 2: Subtract this number from the remaining digits.
- ▶ Step 3: Keep doing this... until you get to a multiple of seven, in which case the original number was perfectly divisible by seven.

For example, to check whether the number 1,904 is divisible by seven, remove the 4, double it to get 8, and subtract that from 190 to get 182. Now remove the 2, double it to get 4, and subtract it from 18 to get 14. Since 14 is divisible by 7, it follows that 1,904 is also divisible by seven.

Question 7: Have a go with these numbers. Stretch your memory skills as you work through the process, visualizing the original numbers changing as you lop off more and more digits. For each one, simply say 'yes' if it's divisible by seven, and 'no' if it isn't.

a) 5,733   b) 24,789   c) 3,946,894

A number is divisible by nine if and only if the sum of its digits is divisible by nine. This little fact is the basis of a number of mathematical 'tricks'.

Here's a nice one. Ask someone to think of a number. It should be at least two digits long, but can be as long as they like. Then get them to reverse the order of the digits to generate a second number. Now ask them to subtract the smaller number from the larger number. From the answer, tell them to choose any digit that is not zero, to keep it secret, but to tell you all the other digits, in any order. Then, with a quick mental calculation, you magically find the missing digit!

So how does it work? Prepare to step deeper into the realms of mathematical thinking... Don't worry if it doesn't make complete sense straight away. This book is going to stretch your understanding of numbers in some new directions, challenging you to grapple with tricky ideas and to see how far your maths mind can go.

The key to this particular trick is that the final number your volunteer arrives at is divisible by nine. That means that the sum of its digits must be divisible by nine. So, when they tell you the digits, all you have to do is to add them up, and calculate how much you need to add to the sum to get to the next multiple of nine. For example, if the digits are 1, 6 and 9, the sum is 16. To get to the next multiple of nine (which is 18) you need to add two – so 2 must be the missing digit.

What about when the sum is already a multiple of nine? In that case the missing digit could be either 0 or 9. That's the reason you have to ask them to choose a digit that *is not zero*: since it can't be zero, the missing digit must be 9.

SO SOMETIMES DIVISION IS NEAT. BUT WHEN IT ISN'T...

Checking the 'reasonableness' of an answer is always important, but in questions of division it's absolutely vital. And here it's not just a matter of checking that the size of the answer looks right. You need to check that your answer *makes sense* in the context of the question you've been set.

This is where your visualization and memory skills are particularly useful. Being able to keep in mind the details of the original question and constantly applying them to the numbers in your head will help you avoid the pitfalls. Ordering 4-seater taxis for a group of 22, you need to be very clear that five and a half taxis will be tricky to arrange. The lift carries 12 people, and there are 39 people needing to get to the top floor. 39 divided by 12 is 3¼. So, what does that mean in the context of passengers and lifts...?

Visualizing the question, working through it in your imagination, focusing on the details and remembering the original context throughout are vital aspects of division in particular, but also very useful thinking skills in general.

Here's a famous division problem that will reveal how well you can now combine calculating skills with *thinking* skills.

Question 8: A shopkeeper was asked how many eggs he'd sold that day. He replied: 'My first customer said he would buy half my eggs, and half an egg more. My second and third customers both said the same thing. And when I'd given them all what they wanted, I was sold out of eggs. What's more, I didn't break an egg all day.' So how many eggs did the shopkeeper sell, *and how did he do it?*

A PIECE OF CAKE

The classic way to think about division is by cutting a cake or a pizza into pieces. But number training pushes you to widen your range of mental models and images, so try imagining we've got a length of cloth to be measured, and a measuring rod. Suppose, for example, that our measuring rod is four units in length, and we want to know how many measuring rods will lie along our length of cloth. If the cloth is 20 units long, then five measuring rods will lie along it, since

$$\frac{20}{4} = 5.$$

What if the cloth is 21 units in length? Well, then we can line up five measuring rods, and we will have one unit of cloth left over: 21 divided by four is five, remainder one. Can we describe this remainder in terms of our measuring rod? It's less than a whole rod, but since it's one unit long, and the rod is four units, we can think of the remainder as a quarter of a rod. So 21 divided by four is five and a quarter, or

$$\frac{21}{4} = 5\frac{1}{4}$$

or, on your calculator, 5.25.

While our intuition is good at handling simple fractions like 1/2 and 1/4, we struggle with more complicated fractions like 18/57 (is this greater or less than 1/3?). Learning to cope provides some excellent training in logical thinking.

The problem with comparing 18/57 and 1/3 is that we're not comparing like with like: on the one hand we have 57ths, and on the other hand, thirds. To decide which of the numbers is bigger, we need to work out how many 57ths there are in one third. Since $57 = 19 \times 3$, we can see that

$$\frac{1}{3} = \frac{19 \times 1}{19 \times 3} = \frac{19}{57}.$$

So 1/3 is the larger fraction. Here it was relatively easy to convert thirds to 57ths, since 57 is divisible by three. But what if our fraction was 18/55? Then we'd have to write both fractions in terms of 165ths ($165 = 3 \times 55$):

$$\frac{1}{3} = \frac{55 \times 1}{55 \times 3} = \frac{55}{165}, \qquad \frac{18}{55} = \frac{3 \times 18}{3 \times 55} = \frac{54}{165}.$$

Decimal notation solves this problem by writing every fraction in terms of tenths, hundredths, thousandths etc. So

$$0.2 = \frac{2}{10} = \frac{1}{5},$$

$$0.25 = \frac{1}{10} + \frac{5}{100} = \frac{25}{100} = \frac{1}{4},$$

$$0.125 = \frac{1}{10} + \frac{2}{100} + \frac{5}{1000} = \frac{125}{1000} = \frac{1}{8}.$$

This shows how to convert from a decimal expression into a fraction. But what about converting from a fraction into a decimal?

Think about 1/4. We're dividing one unit by four. In that unit there are ten tenths. So the number of tenths in 1/4 is 10/4 = 2 1/2. So

$$\frac{1}{4} = \frac{2}{10} + \frac{\frac{1}{2}}{10}.$$

Now we want to divide one tenth by two. In one tenth there are ten hundredths. So the number of hundredths in 1/2 tenth is 10/2 = 5:

$$\frac{\frac{1}{2}}{10} = \frac{\frac{10}{2}}{100} = \frac{5}{100}.$$

And logically…

$$\frac{1}{4} = \frac{2}{10} + \frac{5}{100} = 0.25.$$

Nothing is a problem

You provide an even greater challenge to your logical thinking when you explore how zero fits into this picture.

Imagine first that our length of cloth is zero units long. Then clearly we can line none of our four-unit measuring rods up against it:

$$\frac{0}{4} = 0.$$

No problem so far. But what if our measuring rod is zero units long? Then no matter how many rods we line up, we will never get to a length of 20! It just can't be done.

Mathematicians have struggled with zero ever since it was included as a proper number by seventh-century Indian mathematician Brahmagupta (before then, zero had been thought of only as a place-holder). But zero is not a number like any other. While it's easy to add and subtract zero (both leaving the number unchanged), and multiplying anything by zero gives zero, *dividing* by zero causes problems.

One way out of the conundrum is simply to say that dividing by zero is not allowed; that it's against the rules. If you try to divide a number by zero on your calculator, the chances are that it will give an error. For the most part, simply banning division by zero works OK, but it does seem like a bit of a cop-out.

The twelfth-century Indian mathematician Bhaskara considered division by zero, and suggested that a number divided by zero should be infinite. After all, if we imagine making our measuring rod very small, then lots and lots of copies of it will lie along the length of cloth. As we make it smaller and smaller, we need more and more copies, so that 'in the limit' the number of rods tends to infinity. However, introducing the new number infinity (with the symbol ∞) causes more problems than it solves, since it doesn't obey the usual rules of arithmetic either.

We get into even more trouble when we try to consider dividing zero itself by zero. What should the answer be? We know that zero divided by anything gives zero, that something divided by zero gives infinity, and also that any number divided by itself gives one. So which is it to be?

If we call the answer x, so that

$$\frac{0}{0} = x,$$

then by cross-multiplying we get

$$0 = x \times 0.$$

But since anything times zero is zero, this equation is satisfied no matter what x is. Zero divided by zero can be anything we like! We usually say that 0/0 is undefined. It's probably safest that way…

So dividing by zero is mind-bending, but the principle of division in all its forms provides a range of brain-training opportunities.

Ratios

We're used to seeing ratios in recipes and other instructions ('1 egg for every 100 g of flour', '1 part sand, 2 parts gravel, 3 parts cement') and to hearing them in news reports: 'Tourists now outnumber the residents 3 to 1.' Because the numbers rarely mean *those* numbers, it's particularly important to visualize ratio problems, to focus on the facts, and to think them through in real terms. Like fractions and percentages, ratios reflect changeable situations. In football, if United beat City by a ratio of 3:1, that's not necessarily a final score of 3–1. It just means that, for every goal City scored, United scored 3. Maybe they won 12–4? Ratios require the same logical, balanced thinking we've highlighted throughout this chapter: the 'do the same thing to both' principle.

At the same time, you need to think carefully about the reality of every situation you're exploring and avoid some tempting red-herrings...

Question 9: Marilyn vos Savant includes a great ratio riddle in her book *Brain Power*. Two men were selling neckties. One was offering two for $10 and the other three for $10. Sick of being in competition, they decided to join forces. Each man gave in 30 ties, so they started their new company with a common stock of 60. Since 'two for $10' and 'three for $10' is the same as offering 'five for $20', that's exactly what they decided to do. Now, if the men had continued operating separately, the first man would have earned $150 from his 30 ties at two for $10. The second man would have made $100, based on his 'three for $10' offer. $150 + $100 = $250. So... how come, when their new company has sold all the 60 ties on what seem to be the same terms – five ties for $20 – they've ended up with $240? Where's the missing $10?

Percentages

Question 10: If a shopkeeper decides to increase the price of a £2,000 plasma TV by 20%, but then reduces it by 20% at the end of the day when it hasn't sold... why won't it be priced at £2,000 again?

Percentages are some of the most common fractions we face in day-to-day life.

You need to understand them to work out issues like:

▶ how much you should tip the waiter
▶ why you take home less pay than you actually earn
▶ which mortgage is the best deal
▶ what's going on with your bank account
▶ how you should react to the latest crime figures
▶ whether special offers are really that special.

And percentage problems are great for training your brain.

▶ They challenge you to think on your feet and to choose the best tactic from a range of possible mental methods, often at speed in real-life situations.
▶ They force you to organize your thinking, identifying the key facts and dealing with them efficiently and effectively.

- They strengthen your memory skills, helping you to build up a bank of key percentage facts, and requiring you to visualize and manipulate numbers through various problem-solving processes.
- Percentages are everywhere, offering focused challenges to your mental maths as well as general brain-training opportunities.

Percentages crop up in normal conversation because that's what they're for: to help us compare and contrast numbers and to communicate clearly about what we find. They're a way of untangling complex calculations, and they can be very useful in clarifying your opinions and informing your decisions. But beware: percentages can also tempt you to make dangerous assumptions, and to miss what the numbers actually represent. A layer of common sense in your thinking is more important than ever.

PRACTICAL PERCENTAGES

Percentages appear in many areas of everyday life. Percentages assume that you're dealing with hundredths: dividing a number or amount into a hundred bits.

So 50% means half, 25% is a quarter, 75% three quarters, and 100% the whole... of *anything*. Because, of course, most things don't obviously divide into 100 easy-to-use bits.

So 50% of any pizza, or rugby crowd, or paycheque is half of it. 50% can be huge or tiny: it just depends on the size of the thing in question.

I'll give you 50% of my chips; my co-author is willing to give away 25% of his. The offer you choose depends very much on who has the most chips in the first place. Half is a bigger proportion than a quarter – but half or a quarter of *what*?

So you have to bear in mind what the original amounts are if you're going to make sense of percentage calculations – and make good decisions based on them.

- The murder rate may have gone up by 100%, but if there was only one murder, which then increased to two, that's a very different picture from the town where 25 murders became 50 – but the percentage increase is exactly the same: 100% or 'all again'. *Always be alert to the details and ready to interrogate them.*
- How you respond to a 75% approval rate depends both on the percentage and on the number of people surveyed. Think about

the actual people involved. Does this result refer to three out of four people, 75 out of 100, 6 million out of 8 million…? Small samples can easily give unrepresentative results, and larger surveys offer more robust patterns and trends; but, if approval involved a payment, you could still make lots of money from a small per cent of a large group, or come out badly the other way round. *Always visualize the real information, to help you put it into context and use it to make informed decisions.*

▶ Half of your shampoo bottle may have '50% extra free' splashed all over it, but that really means half of the *usual* amount for free. So if the old 200 ml bottle has grown to 300 ml, you're getting an extra 100 ml: which is nice, but not quite the 150 ml that the package design might suggest. *The brain-training exercises in this book will help you spot the tempting images that don't truly represent the information at hand.*

▶ And what about all that sporting talk of 110% effort? 100% for anyone doing anything means everything they can give. So whether even the most committed competitor can give *more* than that is up to you to decide…

BALANCED BRAINS AGAIN

Once again, an important approach to many percentage calculations is proportional thinking – that common-sense balancing act that uses known facts to help you find the answers you need. With a little practice you can visualize two balanced columns of numbers and quickly fill in any gaps.

If a holiday is going to cost £400, another way to say that is *100% of the holiday costs £400*. Picture the amounts listed side by side.

Percentage	Price
100%	£400

So, keeping the two amounts in proportion, half of the first column, 50%, must be the same as half of the second: £200

Percentage	Price
100%	£400
50%	£200

64

And there are some other easy calculations you can do.

Percentage	Price
100%	£400
50%	£200
10%	£40
1%	£4
15%	15 × £4 = £60

Question 11: See how well you can hold the interim answers in your head to calculate 17.5% of:

a) £440   b) £2,000   c) £68,000

THE SWITCH TRICK

Here's a handy tip to solve many real-life percentage problems. It uses proportional thinking, and the fact that multiplication works 'both ways': that 20 × 50 and 50 × 20 will give you identical answers.

The very useful application of this is that 20% of 50 and 50% of 20 provide the same answer, and the second version is much easier to work out in your head.

Want to calculate 66% of 50 children? Why not switch the numbers to give you 50% of 66. Fifty per cent (half) of 66 is 33.

Need to work out 8% of 200 cars? It should be much easier the other way around. Two hundred per cent of eight (that's 100% of eight, and then 100% of eight again) must be 16.

When you spot 'friendly' numbers, switch round your calculations to make the most of them. Use the key percentage facts to deliver instant answers. Twelve per cent of £75 becomes much more manageable as 75% of £12, which is 3/4 of £12, which is £9.

PERCENTAGE UPS AND DOWNS

In everyday life it's often useful to be able to work out a bit more or a bit less than 100%.

For example: what's 120% of 400? This might be the best way to think of a £400 computer after a 20% price hike. Once again, bring the balanced columns in front of your mind's eye.

Percentage	Amount
100%	400
1%	4
120%	400 + (20 × 4) = 480

And if you'd known the final price but wanted to work it out *without* 20% tax?

Percentage	Amount
120%	480
1%	480 ÷ 120 = 4
100%	4 × 100 = 400

To keep both columns in proportion, whatever you did to the left you'd have to do to the right. Working with 1% on the left meant taking a division step of 120: so you divide the right-hand number by that same amount.

Question 12: It's 20% Day at the jewellery shop, and the sale price of a watch is £160. So what will it cost when the sale is over?

The sale price you're looking at is 80% of the original, so can you calculate 100%?

Percentage	Amount (£)
80%	
1%	
100%	

Question 13: If 60% of a price is £300, what must the whole price be?

And if you need to work out the percentage increase or decrease from the other information you have (for example, the car's gone down in price from £3,000 to £2,400, so what's the percentage drop?) here's what you do.

First, calculate the difference in price. In this case, 3,000 – 2,400 = 600. Then work out what percentage that is of the original price, £3,000. Remember, you can use your understanding of numbers to make this as simple for yourself as possible. 600/3,000 can be simplified to 6/30, which is 1/5. Get the percentage by multiplying that by 100: 1/5 × 100 = 20. The price has dropped by 20%.

Question 14: Use the following questions to practise logical calculating and accurate memory skills.

a) If your salary was £20,000, and you were given a 5% pay rise, what would you now earn?
b) If a bottle of wine increases in price from £8 to £8.50, what's the percentage rise?
c) If a candidate received 30% of the vote, which amounted to 17,100 votes, how many votes were cast in total?
d) Two stores have offers on shampoo. One offers 'buy one, get one half price', while the other offers '30 per cent off'. Which is the better offer?

THE PERCENT CIRCLE

In daily life, there are three key questions about percentages:

▶ What's the ending number? For example, 30% of 70 is what?
▶ What's the starting number? For example, 30% of what is 21?
▶ What's the percentage? For example, What percentage of 70 is 21?

The percent circle is a visualization trick that helps you to cope with all three of these calculations, as well as revealing how the different solving strategies interconnect. It's also useful for number training in general because it shows you more about the relationship between whole numbers, fractions and decimals, and how you can use all three to tackle the trickiest of percentage problems.

The percent circle looks like this:

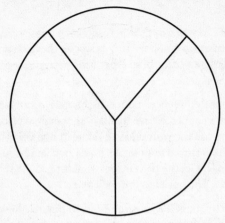

In the three spaces, picture three numbers that make up a percentage statement. For example, 25% of 200 is 50. (Write 25% as a decimal: 0.25, twenty-five hundredths). The result (50) goes at the top, the percentage (0.25) at the left and the starting number (200) slots in on the right.

Authors' insight

To remember what goes where, you could use imagery to 'format' the picture and create powerful reminders. For example, every time you use a percent circle, imagine blue percentage sign wallpaper covering the left segment; a green 'start' button in the right segment; and a bright red equals sign at the top.

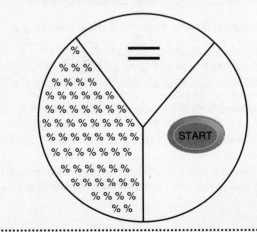

In the example above, the numbers in your percent circle – among all the imagery – would be:

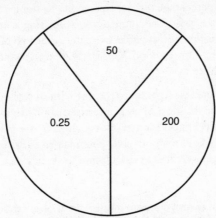

The two crucial features of the percent circle are that:

▶ when you multiply the two numbers at the bottom, the answer is the number at the top
▶ if you make a fraction, with the top number as the numerator and either of the bottom numbers as denominator, that fraction is equal to the other bottom number.

Most percentage puzzles give you two of the numbers. You use your mental imagery to remember where to put them, then the percent circle works its magic to produce the missing number.

What's the ending number?
15% of 30 is…? Picture the numbers in place in the circle. You've got the percentage (in front of the wallpaper on the left) and the starting amount (next to the START button on the right). So the ending number at the big equals sign is simply 0.15 × 30, which is the same as a tenth of 30 and half of that again… 3 and 1.5, 4.5.

What's the starting number?
£90 is 30% of what? This time you're given the percentage on the left and the result at the top. To find the starting number, just imagine a fraction with 90 above 0.3. To work that out, think: what is 90 divided by 0.3? 90 divided by 3 is 30, so dividing it by 0.3 must be ten times bigger, 300, which is the bit you were missing.

What's the percentage?

You're being offered a £30 discount on a carpet that normally costs £120, so what percentage is that? Remember to slot in the offer price, £90, on the right. The number you're missing is on the left; so, like last time, just make a fraction from the other two numbers and calculate the division. 30 ÷ 90. This is 3/9 or 1/3... which is going to be 33.333... per cent.

Put your number-trained brain to the test with the following questions. Make the most of your improved ability to focus on the key facts. Use the logical framework provided by the percent circle, strengthened by your memory skills, but also be as flexible and creative as you can with your calculating strategies.

Question 15:

a) Which deal saves you more money: 30% off a £4,000 holiday or 40% off a £3,000 holiday?

b) The coffee company wants to sell 180 g of beans for the same price as it used to sell 150 g. What percentage giveaway should it advertise?

c) I paid £420 for my new laptop in a '20% off' sale. How much would it have been normally?

Question 16: To round off this chapter, and the first part of the book, here's a famous maths puzzle that should keep you going for a while. Can you use exactly four 4s to make zero and every whole number up to 50? Crucially, you'll need to experiment with decimal points, as well as using +, −, ×, ÷, brackets, square numbers (for example, 4^2), square roots, and the ! sign for 'factorial' (Factorial means the product of all the whole numbers up to and including the number in question; so 4! is $1 \times 2 \times 3 \times 4 = 10$.) Your flexibility with fractions should come in very handy!

Here are a few examples to get you started:

$0 = 44 - 44$
$1 = (4 + 4)/(4 + 4)$
$2 = 4/4 + 4/4$
$3 = (4 + 4 + 4)/4$

Can you do the rest, right up to 50?

NUMBER TRAINING CHALLENGES

1 How balanced is your brain? Practise converting between fractions, decimals and percentages.

   a) Write 0.6 as a percentage
   b) 45% = ?/20
   c) What is 6/25 as a decimal?
   d) What percentage is the same as 'two and three fifths'?

2 Focus on the facts and avoid the traps when you multiply and divide by less than one.

   a) 1/2 × 17   b) 8 ÷ 0.2   c) 1/2 ÷ 1/4   d) 240 × 1/3

3 Use logical divisibility tricks to check whether the following numbers can be divided perfectly by 3, 7 or both.

   a) 179   b) 588   c) 798

4 If your friend spent 1/4 of his life as a boy, 1/5 as a youth, 1/3 as a man, and his remaining 13 years as an old man, how old must he have been when he died?

5 Alice eats 1/3 of a big box of sweets. Bruce then eats 1/3 of the remainder, before Connie eats 1/3 of the rest. That leaves 40 sweets in the box, so how many were there to start with?

6 Visualize the percent circle as you tackle the following questions.

   a) What is 88% of 50?
   b) If 12 of your 20 garden gnomes have been stolen, what percentage have you still got?
   c) 38 is 40% of what?

7 True or false: three successive 5% tax rises make a combined 15% tax rise.

8 Can you transform these binary numbers into an appropriate word?

   100, 1001, 111, 1001, 10100

9 How quickly can you use your knuckles (see 'Extended mind' in the Introduction) to work out the total number of days in June, August and December?

10 Test your memory, concentration and flexible calculating skills as you work through these questions, bringing together all four operations (in the right order...).

a) $27 + 16 \times 12$

b) $180 \div 30 \times 19$

c) $842 - 235 \div 1/2$

d) $180 \times 0.5 + (240 \div 4^2)$

Part two

Thinking about *everything*

5

Shape up your thinking

In this chapter you will learn:
- *the brain-training benefits of thinking about shapes*
- *how numbers can reveal their own shapes, sequences and patterns*
- *tips for winning at spatial games*
- *powerful 3D puzzle-solving skills.*

Thinking about shapes can change your brain. As well as stretching key thinking skills such as visualization and memory, spatial exercises can alter the brain's physical structure. London's black cab drivers were shown to have a larger than average hippocampus – the part of the brain associated with navigation. By doing 'The Knowledge', their rigorous training regime that involves learning and practising thousands of routes around London, it seems that these drivers adapt their brains to suit the particular challenges of their working life.

Puluwat fishermen have a rather different landscape to navigate as they sail their boats among the thousands of islands that make up Micronesia. Over generations they've trained their brains to think about shape and space in a very special way. Using memorized maps of the night sky to guide them, they use their honed visualization skills to imagine that their boats are stationary but the *islands* are moving.

We all use mental pictures to reason about shapes and to prepare ourselves to do things with them physically. We develop thinking skills to help us overcome some tricky challenges. Map-reading and flat-pack furniture assembly, for example, involve some complex mental manipulations, and it can be helpful to visualize the new wardrobe staying in the same place while we rotate around it...

At complicated road junctions a driver will instinctively stop talking, allowing their brain to 'co-ordinate resources'.

Shape and space are challenging concepts, but this chapter shows that we can develop the key skills and learn some useful new strategies. It's also important to understand how spatial thinking can become a powerful tool in itself. We've seen already the importance of using mental models to structure the way we think about maths. Abacus users see the shapes of numbers as they calculate, and they've been shown to have much improved spatial awareness as a result. Learning to handle shapes can improve the way you handle maths in general.

Spatial thinking is at the heart of our place-value, positional number system, and you've seen the importance of holding columns and digits securely in your head. You've also explored arrays, those dot diagrams that help you to understand processes and patterns of numbers by showing you clear evidence of the results. Now you need to focus on numbers that have particularly important shapes. Investigating square and triangular numbers provides some excellent opportunities for training your brain.

Square numbers

We know that $2 \times 2 = 4$, and as an array it forms a square:

Seeing the units arranged like this makes it easier to see why a number multiplied by itself is called a 'square number'.

'3 squared' (written 3^2) is 9:

Exercise your visualization skills by picturing square numbers, starting with 4 and 9 and continuing with 16 (4 × 4), 25 (5 × 5) and so on. Every time you create a square in your mind, focus on what it looks like. Compare it to the square number before it to get a feel for the pattern. Spend a moment thinking about the value of each square array, and imagine stamping each one with its number. Every so often go back through the sequence in your mind. See how far you can go...

Question 1: ... and try to work out the clear pattern within the square number sequence. Without writing anything down, relying only on your imagination, memory and mental maths skills, find a way to predict what the next square number will be.

Ancient Greece

The Greeks were very interested in the shapes of numbers and the patterns they made.

Question 2: Combine a bit of logical and creative thinking. Why was 16 Pythagoras' favourite square? (Taking a walk around it might help...)

Of course Pythagoras was very fond of triangles too... and visualization offers a fantastic way of understanding his most famous theorem: that, in a right-angled triangle, the length of the hypotenuse (the side opposite the right angle) is equal to the sum of the squares of the other two sides.

The classic way to see this is known as Euclid's Proof, from Greece circa 300 BCE. In your mind you construct three squares, using a side of the right-angled triangle to define the size of each one.

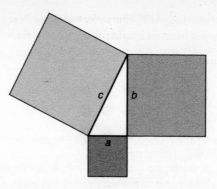

Pythagoras's theorem says that the big square has the same area as the other two together, and that certainly looks right in the picture above; but there are various ways to visualize proof.

The one we'd like you to try involves a bit of splitting, shifting and sliding, but it's a great chance to practise imagining and manipulating shapes as you try to understand them more. We've deliberately included only a few extra details on the diagram below to push you to fill the rest in for yourself.

Imagine the big square split along the dotted line. Now pull at the point shown by the arrow, keeping the corners of the square fixed. The dotted line slides down until it meets the corner of the triangle, pulling the square into two parallelograms.

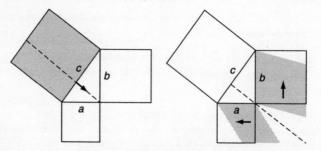

Together, these parallelograms look a bit like an arrowhead – which now moves forwards until it has completely cleared the triangle. If you've done this right, the three back points of the arrowhead should now be the three corners of the original triangle. Finally, the two parallelograms can now split apart, the top one going up, the bottom one down. They still have the same area they started with, but now they can be reshaped into squares: at the top, square *b*, and at the bottom, square *a*.

Pythagorean triples

When the sides of the triangle are all whole numbers they're known as a 'Pythagorean triple' – like 3, 4, 5:

$3^2 + 4^2 = 5^2$ (9 + 16 = 25).

These are beautiful little sets of numbers, and you can use your number-trained brain to find them.

Exercise your focused thinking and memory by using the following method devised by the Alexandrian Greek mathematician Diophantus.

Choose any two numbers – for example, four and 12. Then calculate (and remember):

▶ twice their product (that is, multiply them together and double the answer)
  ▷ 4 × 12 = 48, 48 × 2 = 96
▶ the difference between their squares (multiply each number by itself, then subtract the smaller answer from the larger one)
  ▷ 4 × 4 = 16
  ▷ 12 × 12 = 144
  ▷ 144 − 16 = 128
▶ the sum of their squares
  ▷ 16 + 144 = 160

You should now have three numbers – in this case 96, 128 and 160 – and miraculously these make up a perfect Pythagorean triple:

$96^2 + 128^2 = 160^2$... because 9,216 + 16,384 = 25,600

It's fantastic brain-training to have a go at this in your head, although we recommend you start with small numbers! Even then you'll need to use your thinking skills to the full – especially some of the multiplication tricks from Chapter 3.

Question 3: Work through Diophantus' steps in your head, starting with the numbers two and three. Which Pythagorean triple do you discover?

Triangular numbers

If an array can be reorganized as an equilateral triangle, that number is said to be triangular.

After 1, the sequence of triangular numbers goes like this:

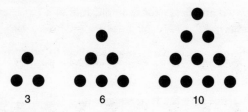

As with square numbers, see how far you can go with this sequence in your mind.

Question 4: See if you can work out a rule for predicting the next triangular number.

Question 5: Can you find a connection between these two sequences: square and triangular numbers?

So the shapes of numbers can help to train your brain, but so too can visible shapes in the world around. Spotting patterns, remembering details, visualizing and manipulating shape and space: these are all vital mental attributes, and you need to seize every chance you get to put them to the test. Many of the thinking skills developed in this book will come in very handy when you're laying a carpet, playing snooker, designing a kitchen, packing a suitcase...

Here's a chance to practise your memory for shapes. Give yourself no more than a minute to study the following design. After that you're going to try to draw it from memory, so make sure you look closely. Spot shapes within shapes; notice any sections that are symmetrical; make a mental note of any parts of the design that remind you of anything; extend your mind by bringing your hands into play, tracing the lines and modelling the design in front of you; and test the theory about talking to yourself, saying aloud all the useful details you want to remember.

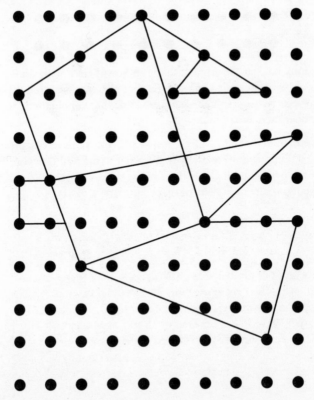

When the time's up, cover the original design and have a go at drawing it from memory on the grid below.

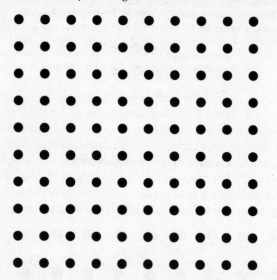

Now look back at the original shape and compare it with your version. Notice the bits you got right, but also think carefully about any aspects that weren't so accurate – and what you might do to remember them next time.

Question 6: In the following challenge, it's your skills of visualization, focused thinking and creativity that are put to the test. Can you make the pyramid using only three of the shapes below it? You're not allowed to rotate or flip any of them.

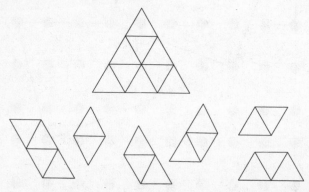

Question 7: This is one of our all-time favourite tests of mental strength. The challenge is to connect all of the nine dots in the grid below, using only four straight lines and without taking your finger off the page. Be as creative as you can – and don't give up, it *can* be done!

Cube nets

Which of the following shapes can be folded up to make a cube?

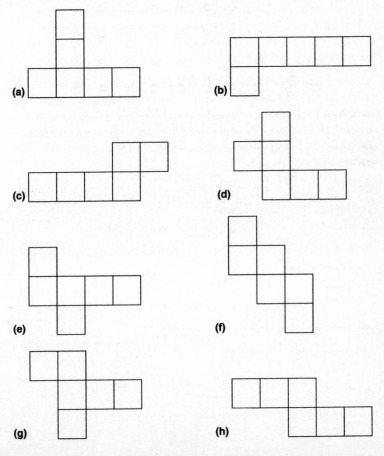

(a)

(b)

(c)

(d)

(e)

(f)

(g)

(h)

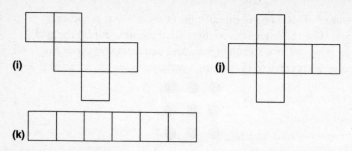

There are 11 different combinations of squares that can be folded to make a cube, but it's not always easy to work out what they are. When they involve four squares in a row you can visualize these being rolled up to form a tube which will be the sides of the cube. Then you need one square on one side for the top, and one on the other side for the bottom: for example, patterns (e) and (j). All together there are six patterns like this. The remaining five foldable patterns are a bit harder to spot.

One way is to think logically. Check if a given shape can be folded into a cube by first making sure it has six squares for the six sides. Then switch on your imagination again, visualize a cube which is painted on one side, and place this cube on one square with the painted side facing down. Now you can imagine rolling the cube around onto each of the other squares in turn, keeping track of the painted side. If the painted side is ever facing down again, then this side will overlap with the starting side when the paper is folded, so it can't make a cube. If you find that no matter which square you start on this never happens, then you know that the shape can be folded to make a cube.

Patterns (a), (b), (c), (d) and (k) can't be folded; the painted squares would overlap.

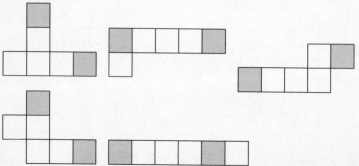

Rotation

How good are you at mentally rotating shapes? Exercise this aspect of your thinking and you might spot improvements in your map-reading, chess-playing or reverse parking. You'll need to concentrate carefully as you study the shape below, then activate all your powers of visualization to draw it *rotated ninety degrees clockwise*. In other words, what would it look like if you gave it a quarter turn to the right?

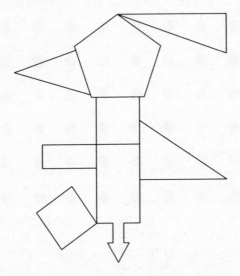

When you've rotated it in your mind, rotate the *page* a quarter turn and see how the two shapes compare.

Reflection

Here's a shape challenge to reflect on... Imagine the dotted line is a mirror and try drawing in the reflection of the top design.

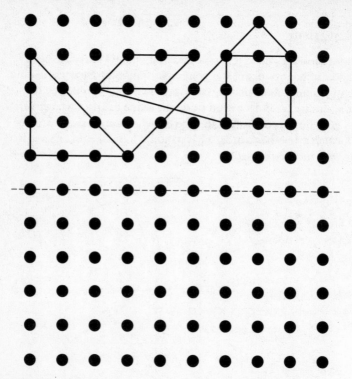

Question 8: If you draw around the reflection of your face in a steamed-up bathroom mirror, the area of the shape you've drawn will be exactly half that of your real face. Why?

The more you train your brain to cope with shapes, the more observant you'll be about shapes in the world around you. Be inquisitive, focus on details, ask why particular shapes are used.

Question 9: Visualize an electricity pylon. You've seen these many times in the real world, but, by using your memory and looking with your mind's eye, can you pick out the key shape that's used to form these structures? Pylons are constructed by joining together lots of this shape. What is it – and why is it so useful?

Rubik's Cube

Stretch your spatial skills – and your thinking skills in general – by exploring how mathematicians tackle the Rubik's Cube. As you'd probably guess, they have their own particular way of getting their heads around a challenge like this.

As with most 3D puzzles, the Rubik's Cube can be described by what mathematicians call a *state space* – the set of all possible configurations of the cube – and a *set of moves* which describes how to move from one state to another. The goal is to get from the 'initial configuration' (probably jumbled up) to another chosen configuration (solved, presumably) using only the allowed moves (in this case, without peeling the stickers off!)

The difficulty is that the basic moves change the configuration a lot. Just as you move one piece into place, another two are moved out of place...

One way to tackle the Rubik's Cube is to work out *combinations* of moves that don't change the configuration too much. You can see how this works by focusing on what happens to one side of the cube.

To show how a combination of simple moves can be put together to create a *compound move*, let's start with the cube in its completed configuration and carry out a series of four moves.

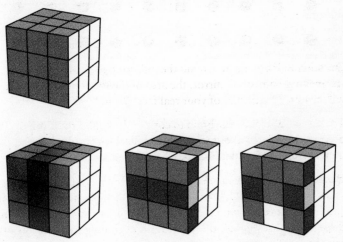

Challenge yourself to picture what happens in your mind's eye. First, move the middle backwards. Then...

▶ turn the front anticlockwise
▶ move the middle forwards
▶ turn the front clockwise.

These are really two moves and then the opposite two moves.

So what's happened to the top face? Can you visualize it now?

It looks like this:

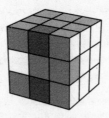

While each individual move affects three of the top squares, your series of four moves has extracted just one of the top squares and left the remaining eight in place. Performing that series in reverse would create a compound move and let you insert a square into the correct position on the top face while leaving all the others unchanged.

> **Authors' insight**
>
> Have a go yourself. Get hold of a Rubik's Cube and experiment with different combinations of twists and turns to see how they might come together as effective compound moves. If you decide you're going to beat the Rubik's cube World Record, you'll need to get your time down to well below ten seconds. And if your powers of visualization are strong enough, why not try doing it blindfolded? The current record for that is just over 30 seconds!

Question 10: Practise your estimation skills. How many different configurations of a Rubik's Cube do you think there are?

NUMBER TRAINING CHALLENGES

1 Picture a six-storey cannonball pile, with the balls packed as efficiently as possible.

   How many balls does it hold?

2 Study the shape below for one minute, then draw it from memory – rotated 90 degrees anticlockwise.

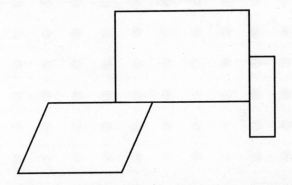

3 If you put your arm through a long loop of string, then put your hand in your jacket pocket, how could you remove the loop without removing your hand?

4 Test your ability to visualize and manipulate shapes. Study this design, then cover it up and try drawing its *reflection* in the bottom half of the grid.

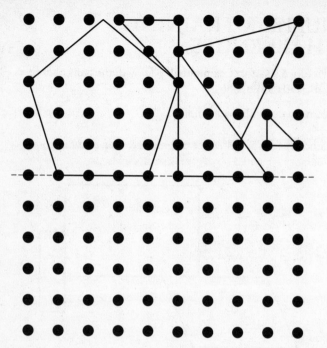

5 How could you cut a hexagonal slice from a perfect cube of cheese?

6 Imagine a wooden cube measuring 3 cm × 3 cm × 3 cm. How many cuts would your need to divide it into 27 cubes measuring 1 cm by 1 cm?

7 What's the sum of the first ten square numbers?

8 Calculate 30% of 50, plus 3/8 of 160, multiplied by nine, divided by five, divided by ten, subtract half of 17 – then square the answer and multiply by the square root of 16.

9 Can you remember how to multiply by 11 in your head? To solve the following questions, use the logical system explained in Chapter 3 and strengthen your memory, concentration and attention to detail.

   a) 89 × 11   b) 237 × 11   c) 4,952 × 11

10 Can you find the creative way to cut a cake into eight equal pieces with only three knife cuts?

6

Measurable improvements

In this chapter you will learn:
- *how to improve your ability to estimate*
- *tips and tricks for a variety of measuring challenges*
- *new ways to read and represent data*
- *how calculating with pi can sharpen your brain.*

We've always been interested in measuring the world – and then finding ways to let others see what we've discovered.

We start by measuring ourselves. What child doesn't love recording their height against the doorframe? Our first units of measurement tend to be our hands and other body parts, allowing us to perform useful comparisons and calculations. After that we start experimenting with objects around us, then move on to using

Names in numbers: Eratosthenes

Back in 300 BCE, the Greek mathematician Eratosthenes worked out the circumference of the Earth and the distance to the sun, basing his calculations on the length of stadiums or *stades*. He was able to present people with statistics that meant something to them, achieving a remarkable degree of accuracy in the process and using his discoveries to powerful effect. He invented a system for longitude and latitude and introduced the world to the idea of geography. A millennium and a half before the right technology was invented, Eratosthenes found ways to use the thinking tools at his disposal to achieve phenomenal feats of measurement.

whatever standard systems we're shown. Experience helps us to develop a sense of length, weight, time… and as the rest of our maths skills strengthen, we learn how to handle the measurement data we collect: to examine, apply and communicate it effectively.

The examples and exercises in this chapter will continue to develop all your key thinking skills and present more opportunities to put them to use. Along the way you may meet a few unfamiliar methods of data-handling, ramping up the challenge to your maths brain and extending your number training in some intriguing new directions.

Authors' insight

We're not very good at trusting our own instincts about measures. In one experiment, people were asked to try on shoes which, unknown to them, had been labelled wrongly by a size in either direction. Despite the shoes themselves fitting perfectly, the shoppers showed a distinct reluctance to buy them, trusting the size on the box rather than their own perceptions.

Estimation

Honing your estimation skills is very good brain training.

- ▶ If you have a temperature readout on your car dashboard, get into the habit of predicting what it will say every morning before you turn the key.
- ▶ Reset the trip-counter and see how accurately you can estimate the distance you've travelled when you arrive at your destination.
- ▶ Estimate the weight of fresh produce in the supermarket and then weigh it to see how close you came.
- ▶ Guess the age of your favourite sports stars, actors or politicians, then use the internet to check your success.

Question 1: How old are the following famous people? Combine attention to detail with instinct, general knowledge, and confidence in your perceptions. For each name below, estimate the year in which they were born.

a) Madonna   b) Daniel Radcliffe   c) Venus Williams   d) Tony Blair

Question 2: Picture a tin of Heinz beans. How many beans are inside? It's an image that almost anyone can visualize, and most of us also have the experience of opening, cooking and eating the beans to help us arrive at our answer. After your first guess, see what a bit of careful self-questioning can do to pin down your best final estimate.

Units of measurement

You can use some simple memory techniques to help you retain important details about measuring units. For example, it's useful to know which is bigger: miles or kilometres, pounds or kilograms, metres or yards – so make sure you visualize the bigger unit in bigger writing. Picture the pairs of measure in your mind's eye and exaggerate the word MILE next to kilometre, KILOGRAM by pound and METRE alongside yard. Remembering the bigger unit will help you when you start to compare and convert amounts.

Make sure you know what a few benchmark measures look or feel like. Most of the time you don't have to carry out complex conversions; you just need some useful mental models and images to help you make sensible decisions.

A one-person bag of crisps typically weighs 30 g. A can of fizzy drink holds 330 ml. A school ruler is 30 cm long. An episode of *The Simpsons* is on TV for half an hour.

Sometimes you should try cooking without measuring out any of the ingredients. Spend a day free from watches and clocks. Reactivate your instinctive ability to make good judgements about real-life measurements.

When you do need to calculate accurate conversions between different units, use your memory again to store a few key facts. You can also use the extended mind principle here to boost your chances of success.

1 inch = 2.54 centimetres

The distance from the tip of your thumb to its knuckle is close to an inch. Look at that bit of your body and imagine seeing three digits tattooed onto the skin there – in pictures. The 2 could be a swan, the 5 a hook, and the 4 the mast of a sailing boat. Pictures are usually much easier to remember than numbers. You could even turn the pictures into a scene or story and imagine it being played out on that inch-long bit of your thumb: maybe a swan using a hook to winch a yacht out of the water. So the digits here are 2, 5 and 4 – and your general knowledge should be enough to tell you that this conversion is 2.54 cm to one inch.

1 mile = 1.6 kilometres

What's roughly a mile from your house? Picture this building, landmark, or village and fix another memorable image in place there, based on the digits 1 and 6 (and a decimal point in between). Maybe they look to you like a long matchstick and a cannon. Or a pen and a musical note. The decimal point in the middle could be the broken top of the matchstick lying next to the cannon, or an inkblot from the pen you're using to write out some sheet music. What funny, strange, rude or otherwise memorable imagery will remind you of 1.6, which is the number of kilometres to every mile?

Here are three more useful conversion facts. For each one, think carefully about the real-world imagery that might give you a place to start, then be creative with the shape of the numbers to build some memorable clues into your brain.

1 yard = 0.91 metres

1 kilogram = 2.2 pounds

1 litre = 1.76 pints

CLEVER CONVERSIONS

You can also use some of the tips and tricks you've learned so far to help with converting measurements. When you're converting from inches to centimetres, it's useful to think of 1 inch being roughly 2.5 cm; but going from cm to inches it may be easier to think of 10 cm being the same as 4 inches.

To convert kilograms to pounds you need to multiply by 2.2. You can do this most easily in two steps: first double, then add another 10%. So 45 kg is 99 lbs (double 45 is 90, 10% of 90 is 9, 90 + 9 = 99).

A similar trick works when converting pints to litres – if you only need a rough answer. One pint is 0.568 litres, which is approximately 0.55 litres. So to convert from pints to litres, divide by 2 and then add 10%. Twenty pints, for example, is about 11 litres (half of 20 is ten, 10% of ten is 1, 10 + 1 = 11), which isn't far from the exact conversion: 11.36 litres.

Question 3: You have two unmarked containers: one carries exactly three litres, the other two litres – but you need to measure out one litre. Can you think of two ways to do it?

And to reveal how data-handling goes beyond graphs and pie charts, here's an insight into how a number-trained brain might tackle a measuring problem like this. By choosing the most appropriate way to analyse your data, you can arrive at the specific answers you need, but also prove some more general theories about what's going on.

Suppose you have a three-pint jug and a five-pint jug, and you want to measure out four pints. Is it possible? And if it is, how do you do it?

Start with both jugs empty and fill up the five-pint jug. A useful way to record this would be (5,0), showing that the five-pint jug has five pints in it, and the three-pint jug is empty, and giving you a neat pair of figures.

Next you can fill the three-pint jug from the five-pint jug. You can write this as (2,3), since two pints remain in the five-pint jug, and three pints are now in the three-pint jug. Empty the three-pint jug, which corresponds to (2,0), and then pour the water left in the five-pint jug into the three-pint jug (0,2). Now fill the five-pint jug again, to give (5,2). Finally fill the three-pint jug from the five-pint jug. Since only one more pint will fit in the three-pint jug, there are four pints left in the five-pint jug: (4,3).

It's quite complicated to keep all this in your head, so the pairs of numbers showing how many pints there are in each jug should help your memory to stay on track. But you can do even better if you graph the numbers. The diagram here shows that you could draw up a chart with the volume of water in the five-pint jug on the horizontal axis, and the volume of water in the three-pint jug on the vertical axis.

Then each combination of volumes in the five- and three-pint jugs corresponds to a point on the chart.

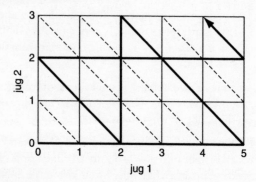

You can fill or empty the five-pint jug, which corresponds to moving horizontally; or fill or empty the three-pint jug, which corresponds to moving vertically; or empty the contents of one jug into the other, which corresponds to moving along diagonal lines. Crucially, since there are no measurements on the jugs, you can only stop when the jugs are either empty or full: in other words, only at the boundary of the chart.

To measure four pints you just 'bounce' around the chart, crossing from one edge to another until you reach the volume you want. If you ever get back to where you started – without reaching the desired volume – then you know it can't be done.

Question 4: Thinking flexibly, you could also have started by filling the three-pint jug. Have a go at finding the pairs of numbers this would produce. Try to imagine how they'd look on the chart, then compare your version of this alternative approach with the diagram at the end of the chapter.

Money maths

Question 5: Here's a quick challenge to get you thinking about monetary measures. In US currency, changing the ten-cent piece to 18 cents, and the 25-cent coin to 29 cents, would make change-giving a more efficient procedure. Giving change to a dollar, the average number of coins required would drop from 4.7 to 3.9. In the UK, to make any amount up to £5, the average number of coins required at the moment is 4.6. Adding two new coins into the system – a 133-pence and a 137-pence coin – would reduce this average – but by how much? As always, use all your thinking skills to make your estimate as accurate as possible.

Pi

The number 3.1415926... is important in the world of measuring – and maths in general. It relates to circles: the ratio of any circle's circumference to its diameter. It's a very powerful number because its decimal representation never ends or gets stuck in a repeating pattern. The number known as *pi* – π – has intrigued people for thousands of years.

The Babylonians and Ancient Egyptians were using fractions very similar to pi from about 1900 BCE. Archimedes (287–12 BCE) was the first person to measure it rigorously. Computers have now listed pi to more than a trillion decimal places – although 39 will probably do. That's all a physicist needs to draw a circle the size of the observable universe and to make it accurate to the size of a hydrogen atom!

Using pi, you can work out the circumference, diameter and area of a circle even when you don't know all the measurements. It's a useful practical tool in art, design, clothes-making, DIY and so on.

For example:

Circumference (C) = 2πr (2 × π × the radius, or half the diameter). If your circle has a radius of 10 cm, its circumference must be 2 × π × 10, which comes to 62.83 cm.

Area $(A) = \pi r^2$ (the radius multiplied by itself and then multiplied by π). Using the same circle, r × r = 100, and π × 100 = 314.2, giving an area of 314.2 cm²

Diameter $(D) = C / \pi$ (the circumference divided by π). If the circumference is 62.83 cm, divide that by π and you get 20 cm.

Question 6: Exercise your logic and flexible thinking by explaining how you could work out the area of a circle if all you knew was its circumference.

Question 7: A pizza company sells small (diameter 9", price £6.95), medium (diameter 13", price £10.95) and large (diameter 15", price £14.95) pizzas. Calculate a price per square inch for each size. Which is the best value?

Many calculators now have a π button, and of course you can approximate pi to a manageable number like 3.142. But it's very good number training to try *learning* this fascinating number – at least some of it...

REMEMBERING PI

Memorizing pi has been a remarkably popular pursuit over the years and the world record is hotly contested. Lu Chao from China took more than 24 hours to recite pi to 67,890 decimal places without a single error. Akira Haraguchi of Japan, a number memorizer with a proven track record, has recently submitted a claim for 100,000 digits.

Haraguchi's technique is to convert numbers into letters and words in his mind so that he can turn them into memorable stories. It requires great imagination, extreme attention to detail and deep concentration – which is why it could be good for *your* brain to give it a go!

One straightforward technique is to use the length of words to represent the digits of pi. So, to remember the first seven decimal places, you could learn this sentence:

> *How I wish I could calculate pi.*

The word lengths here are 3,1,4,1,5,9 and 2 letters... giving you the first seven digits of pi.

The next example is popular with students:

> *How I like a drink, alcoholic of course,*
>
> *after the heavy lectures involving quantum mechanics.*

Remember that sentence and you know pi to 15 places.

Have a go yourself. Read the following mnemonic poem out loud. After each line, close your eyes and go back through the words in your mind, quickly calculating the number of letters in each one and calling them out. This strange verse takes pi to 20 decimal places.

> *Now... I wish I could recollect pi.*
>
> *'Eureka,' cried the great inventor.*
>
> *Christmas Pudding, Christmas Pie*
>
> *Is the problem's very centre.*

Question 8: Read the poem aloud three times – then cover it up while you try to answer these questions from memory.

a) What is the 16th number of pi after the decimal point?
b) In this particular slice of pi... what comes after 592?
c) How many times does the number 5 appear in the first 20 decimal places?

NUMBER TRAINING CHALLENGES

1 Imagine you've bought eight professional juggling balls of identical size and weight, only to hear that a mistake has been made and one of the balls is in fact slightly heavier than the rest. Rather than sending them all back to the supplier, can you design a step-by-step process to identify the 'bad' ball? All you have to help you is a simple set of balancing scales. It's possible to solve this problem in just two weighings. Can you work out how?

2 Put your memory skills to the test by learning the first 31 digits of pi. Read this poem aloud several times, stick it on your fridge, make it into a bookmark... give yourself time to get to know it, then see if you can use the word lengths to give you the numbers you need.

Sir, I bear a rhyme excelling
In mystic force, and magic spelling
Celestial sprites elucidate
All my own striving can't relate
Or locate they who can cogitate
And so finally terminate.
Finis.

3 Use everything you learned in this chapter to estimate the answers to the following questions.

   a) How many CDs do you own?
   b) What's your car's current mileage?
   c) How many words are there in this book?

4 You've got an open barrel of beer and want to know whether it's more or less than half full. How could you do it, without the help of any measuring implements – other than your brain?

5 You have a balance and five items with known weights: a small coin weighing 5 g, a pen weighing 10 g, a pencil-sharpener weighing 20 g, a hole-punch weighing 40 g and a stapler weighing 80 g. How many different possible weights can you measure with these items? See if you can spot the cleverest way to work this out.

6 Use the tricks explained in this chapter – and all the thinking skills you've developed so far – to help you with the following conversions.

   a) How many centimetres are there in 16 inches?
   b) Convert 20 kg into pounds.
   c) 32 pints is roughly... how many litres?
   d) How many millimetres make 100 km?

7 How many 8 cm lengths could you cut from a ribbon measuring 11.3 m?

8 What is 45% of 185 litres?

9 You know how to multiply two two-digit numbers. So, can you visualize, estimate and then calculate the area of a mat measuring 57 cm by 31 cm?

10 Three tennis balls fit exactly into a cylindrical container. Which is larger: the height of the container, or the circumference of the rim?

7

Chances to shine

In this chapter you will learn:
- *why probabilities can be so perplexing*
- *the challenge of analysing averages*
- *backwards thinking to reverse the odds*
- *winning strategies for probability games.*

Probability is one of the most challenging areas of everyday maths, and we can blame evolution. Our brains just aren't designed to cope with it.

Evolution is about survival, and we evolved our perception of probability to help us survive rare but catastrophic events. We're good at spotting them and they loom large in our minds. When you hear a news report about a plane crash, it's hard not to worry more about your up-coming holiday flight. It just seems more likely that a similar fate will happen to you. Statistically, of course, you're far more likely to meet your end during the car journey to the airport, and then when you're walking across the car-park... We just instinctively over-estimate the likelihood of rare but dramatic events.

We're much better when it comes to estimating things that aren't quite so 'life and death', and when we know we're going to get several chances. We can handle things we can see and count. How often will you pass a red car on the way to get your plane? What are the chances of the next song on the radio being your favourite? These are probability questions you can answer with much more accuracy. If the next car isn't red, or that particular song hasn't come up yet, there'll be another chance in a minute and your original prediction will probably even out somewhere along the line. But when you're considering possible plane crashes, probability is a much less manageable concept, and it's much harder for your brain to maintain useful perspective – especially after the news story you heard over breakfast.

In fact, emotions play a major role in our problems with probability. We're easily confused by the potential impact of something happening or not. When you're buying your lottery ticket, are you really thinking accurately about your chances of winning? We're all too easily misled by tempting theories. 'Black's come up ten times now on the roulette wheel. Surely red has to come up next?' And, as these two examples show, so many of the situations in which probability is important to us are, well, *important to us*: about winning and losing, getting sunshine on your wedding day, finding your lost ring, getting caught, getting pregnant, getting better…

This chapter shows how important it is to understand something about the maths of chance, but also to have the mental agility to cope with the big thinking challenges it presents. Probability questions provide some excellent opportunities to experiment with new ways of thinking, often going against your instincts. More than ever you need to know the mental strategies that will let you calculate, check and apply probability confidently in a range of brain-stretching ways.

Names in numbers: Gottfried Wilhelm Leibniz

Leibniz, born in Germany in 1646, was an influential mathematician and philosopher. He set himself an ambitious target: to use mathematical rules to make every decision clear. His system involved visualizing rectangles. The length of one side represented the amount of 'goodness' aimed at; the other, the likelihood of the decision paying off as planned. So very good things that were very likely to happen produced very big rectangles in Leibniz's mind, and a clear incentive to pursue that line of action – in stark visual contrast to small rectangles representing less potential good and less chance of happening. We'll see in this chapter that using visualization can certainly help to tackle complex questions of chance, even if applying definitive calculations to an uncertain world is never as easy as Leibniz might have hoped.

Question 1: This puzzle is one of the most famous probability questions ever. It's become known as the Monty Hall problem, after the host of *Let's Make A Deal!*, the US game-show which featured the following scenario.

A valuable prize has been hidden behind one of three doors. You start your hunt for the prize by choosing one of the doors. The host, who knows where the prize is, now opens one of the other two doors (showing that the prize is not there), and then offers you the chance to change. So, you've now got a choice between just two doors, and you know that one of them hides the prize you're after. The question is: does it make sense to change your original guess?

This puzzle has provoked a great deal of controversy over the years. Many eminent thinkers have argued the case for and against changing. The answer has now been clearly established, and – like many in this area of maths – it's a surprising one. Yes: by changing your choice, you significantly improve your chance of winning the prize. Can you explain why?

The Monty Hall problem shows that a number-trained brain needs to be able to challenge intuition with mathematical analysis. We've seen that creativity can be a powerful problem-solving skill; but, in questions of probability, logic is particularly important. Without it, our hopes, fears and personal prejudices can all too easily get in the way.

Authors' insight

In Lake Wobegone, the fictional Minnesota town created by writer Garrison Keillor, *all* the children are 'above average', and the locals are predictably satisfied with this state of affairs. The 'Lake Wobegone effect' has been written about since in many different contexts. In a study of a million American high school students, 70% regarded themselves as having above-average leadership skills. Another report claimed that more than 80% of us believe we're above-average drivers.

In the UK, there were calls for the education system to be improved when 50% of students were said to be below average. But is it even possible for more than 50% of students to be above average? The answer is no, and yes.

See if you can get your head around these ideas. The *median* average of a set of data tells you the halfway point, and there are exactly 50% of student test results above the median and 50% below. But the *mean* average of a set of test results is different. To find the mean you add up all the scores and divide by the number of entrants. The mean is the mark that everybody would have got if they all got the same mark and the total score was unchanged.

So, if there are ten students sitting a test and their scores are 70,70,70,70,70,70,70,70,70,100, then the average is 73, and 90% of the students are below average!

On the other hand, if the scores are 70,70,70,70,70,70,70,70,70,40, then the average is 67, and this time 90% are *above* average.

Authors' insight
If you want to get more people above the average, then you have to make sure that there are a few really bad students, and no really good ones!

The law of averages

You toss a coin ten times and it comes up heads eight times and tails twice. Do you think it's more likely to come up heads or tails next time?

On average, there should be the same number of heads as tails. Since tails are currently behind, there's a natural instinct that says the coin should land on tails more frequently in the future in order to 'catch up'.

There are many Roulette 'systems' that are based on this idea. In a typical example, the player keeps a record of the colour of the number that the roulette wheel stops on. If a run of six reds comes up in a row, the player places a stake on black for the next spin. Or perhaps he waits until the total number of reds is ten more than the total number of blacks and then bets black. Somehow the idea is that the wheel knows it has to balance the numbers of reds and blacks.

Of course the law of averages is true: it does indeed say that on average you would expect the same number of heads as tails, the same number of blacks as reds. But it's also true that the chances of heads or tails on the next toss are still 50:50. How can both of these statements be true?

Probabilities throw up some mind-bending ideas. It's useful to understand the maths and to have some practical strategies for real-life situations; but grappling with probabilities is also a great way to challenge and exercise a wider range of thinking skills.

The key here is to realize that the law of averages applies *on average*; and to have the imagination to cope with some very large-scale experiments.

If we make a lot of tosses, roughly half will be heads – and the two key words here are *a lot* and *roughly*. If we make another thousand tosses, the advantage that heads currently has becomes swamped by the number of new heads and tails we count. If we make another million tosses, the results of the ten tosses we've already made become insignificant. This is what the law of averages says. It doesn't matter how big a lead heads currently has because, if we make enough tosses in the future, that lead will fade into the noise and have a very small effect on the average.

The word 'average' seems to imply something very negative, so it's no wonder that we're reluctant to apply it to ourselves, to believe that we're 'typical' in any way. The following game demonstrates this, and provides an opportunity to develop some important thinking skills.

D.I.Y. LOTTERY

Here's how it works. Everyone picks a whole number, writes it down but keeps it secret. When the choices are finally revealed, the winning player is the one who picked the lowest unique number.

Most people simply don't accurately assess the strategy involved. We find it hard to believe that someone else will choose the same low number as us, and set our 'ceiling' too low. Research shows that we tend to set a horizon of around 20, or roughly twice the number of players. But reassess the situation, stretch your parameters a little, and you might be surprised how often you win – as your opponents cancel each other out with their identical ideas.

Thinking about probability

There are two distinct ways of looking at probabilities. Flex your mental muscles now to consider them both.

PROBABILITIES AS EVENTS/TOTAL EVENTS

If I throw a die, what's the probability that the result will be a three? Clearly the answer is one chance in six. Mathematicians express probability in terms of fractions (or decimals, or percentages). So one chance in six is written as a probability of 1/6. As a decimal this is about 0.16; as a percentage it's about 16 per cent.

> **Authors' insight**
> A bookmaker would look at this situation slightly differently, expressing the chance in terms of odds of 5 to 1 *against*: that is, there are five negative outcomes for every positive outcome.

But how did we come up with the answer 1/6? Well, there are six faces on the die, and only one of these is a three, so we can calculate the chance of getting a three as

$$\frac{\text{number of outcomes leading to a three}}{\text{total number of possible outcomes}}$$

This method of calculating probabilities assumes that all the possible outcomes are equally likely to occur. Of course, that's exactly what we hope with the throw of a die or the toss of a coin, but in some cases we need to be careful to make sure the assumption is correct (for example, it's *not* true that a person is as likely to be born on the first of the month as on the 31st, since all 12 months have a first day, but only seven months have 31 days).

From this definition of probability we can see that a probability is always a number between zero and one. Zero represents an event that will never happen (there are no successful outcomes), while a probability of one says that an event will always happen (the number of successful outcomes is the same as the total number of outcomes – so every outcome must be successful).

		Roll of first die					
		1	2	3	4	5	6
Roll of second die	1	2	3	4	5	6	7
	2	3	4	5	6	7	8
	3	4	5	6	7	8	9
	4	5	6	7	8	9	10
	5	6	7	8	9	10	11
	6	7	8	9	10	11	12

Much more of a challenge to your number-trained brain is to consider the roll of *two* dice, and to work out the chance of rolling a particular total.

From the table you can see that there are 36 possible outcomes. This is a key rule in probability calculations:

If there are *a* possible outcomes for one event, and *b* possible outcomes for another (independent) event, then there are *a* × *b* possible outcomes for the two events combined.

Of these 36 outcomes, there are six that lead to a score of seven (you could do it by throwing 1-6, 2-5, 3-4, 4-3, 5-2 or 6-1). So the chance of rolling a total of seven is 6/36, or 1/6.

Question 2: Strengthen your concentration and attention to detail by studying the information above and completing the following table.

Total	2	3	4	5	6	7	8	9	10	11	12
Number of ways to make it	1	2	?	?	?	?	?	?	?	?	?
Probability	1/36	1/18	?	?	?	?	?	?	?	?	?

Authors' insight

The next time you play Monopoly – or any other two-dice game – give your brain some useful exercise. Before each throw, think about the numbers you want – and *don't* want – to come up, and work out the chances in your head. Start basing your tactics on the mathematical odds. The dice may still surprise you, but great game-players make probability a key part of their strategy for success.

PROBABILITIES AS FREQUENCIES

There's another way of thinking about probabilities: in terms of the *relative frequency* of certain events happening. For example, you could think of the probability of rolling a three with a single die as the number of times three comes up *on average*. You could then calculate this probability 'experimentally' by rolling a die lots of times and keeping a running total of the number of threes rolled.

The probability of rolling a three could be defined as:

$$\text{probability of rolling a } 3 = \frac{\text{number of 3s rolled}}{\text{total number of rolls}}$$

Of course, this definition of probability only works if the total number of rolls is large. (In fact, it really only holds as the number of rolls becomes infinite, because otherwise there will always be a small error.)

Maths on drugs

Maybe this gives us a more accurate idea of probability because it works even if the die isn't fair. It's a common method in the real world (rather than the theoretical maths realm of dice and coins). For example, this is the main method used to assess the effectiveness of drugs in clinical trials.

Roughly speaking, the probability of a drug benefiting any patient is the number of patients who benefited in a clinical trial divided by the total number of patients in the trial.

It's also the approach used in weather reports. When the weather presenter says that there's a ten per cent chance of rain, this means that when the scientists ran their weather prediction models on the computer with slight variations in the parameters, for every ten simulations they performed, one resulted in rain.

Question 3: If the forecaster says there's a 50% chance of it raining on Saturday, and a 50% chance of it raining on Sunday, are we guaranteed rain over the weekend?

Reverse odds

There's a creative thinking tactic that can help when calculating probabilities. It's similar to the 'backwards thinking' approach so useful for solving number puzzles and handling fractions. It's a good example of the benefits that come from taking a mental step back from a problem, allowing you to see the whole picture and to use all the facts at your disposal.

It begins with a question like: what's the probability that I *don't* throw a three with a single roll of a die? If I don't roll a three, that means I must roll a one, two, four, five or six. That's five chances of success out of six possible outcomes, so the odds are five in six and the probability 5/6.

And you can use the sort of 'balanced thinking' that's been cropping up throughout this book by adding together the 'will' and 'won't' probabilities. The probability of rolling a three, added to the probability of not rolling a three, equals one, because

$$\frac{1}{6} + \frac{5}{6} = 1.$$

This is true in general for any two outcomes that can't both happen – you can't roll a three and not roll a three at the same time! – and which together make up the whole range of possible outcomes: either rolling a three or not. In a mathematician's mind it becomes a law:

probability of A + probability of NOT A = 1.

This law is amazingly useful, since there are many times when the probability of an event happening is difficult to calculate, but the probability of it *not* happening is much easier to find.

In all issues of probability it's more important than ever to focus on the facts. You need to isolate the key details and use them to define the exact situation in question.

Combining probabilities

Suppose we roll two dice again, but now instead of adding the totals we ask for the probability that the first shows a one *and* the second shows a three. The chance of this happening is clearly one in 36, because we know that there are 36 possible outcomes, and only one of them is 1-3. There's a 1/6 chance of getting number 1 on the first die, 1/6 of getting 3 on the second – and, since the rolls are *independent*, we just multiply the two fractions together to get the probability of a 1-3 result: 1/36.

Question 4: Test your logical thinking by applying this rule to the following scenario. In a game involving dice being thrown and coins being tossed, you can win on your next go if you roll a six and toss a head. What are the chances of that happening?

It's good for your number training to make things even more complicated. Focus on the facts, keep using visualization to picture the dice, coins, balls in bags or whatever, and strengthen your logical thinking as you build the rules of probability into your brain.

Let's go back to the roll of two dice. We can combine probabilities in another way. Instead of asking for the probability that you roll a one with the first die *and* a three with the second, you can work out the chances of rolling a one with the first die *or* a three with the second. Since you're combining your chances, adding is the right approach – but there's an important pitfall to spot. Pay great attention to the details now and see if you can see it.

The probability of the first die showing a one is 1/6, and you do need to combine that with the probability of the second die showing a three, which is also 1/6.

But, the answer is not 2/6. Why not? Give yourself time to explore what's happening in your mind...

The problem is that you've counted something twice. This is why attention to detail is such an important thinking skill. You've practised it with tally marks and percentage problems... and now it's time to do so with probabilities.

In a question like this, if you're not careful, you double-count the outcome in which the first die shows a one and the second shows a three. It was part of the first 1/6 and part of the second 1/6, but you can't count it twice. So, as a simple remedy, just take off 1/36 to make up for the double counting and restore the balance:

probability of 1 with first or 3 with second $= \dfrac{1}{6} + \dfrac{1}{6} - \dfrac{1}{36} = \dfrac{11}{36}$.

		Roll of first die					
		1	2	3	4	5	6
Roll of second die	1	2	3	4	5	6	7
	2	3	4	5	6	7	8
	3	4	5	6	7	8	9
	4	5	6	7	8	9	10
	5	6	7	8	9	10	11
	6	7	8	9	10	11	12

It's always a good idea to look for other evidence that you're right. Number training is about having a range of strategies to strengthen your accuracy. In this case, you might take a look at the table of outcomes – and see that, out of the 36 possible outcomes, 11 satisfy the criteria. The table also makes it clear that the 1-3 box is counted twice when you add up the probabilities of a one with the first die and a three with the second.

So the rules for combining probabilities (for independent events) are:

probability of A and B = probability of A × probability of B

probability of A or B = probability of A + probability of B – probability of A and B.

Question 5: Test your memory, logic and flexible thinking with the following probability problems. Push your brain to visualize the events, incorporating 'common sense' into your calculations as well as relying on the logic and laws of maths.

a) For a pair of dice, what's the probability of rolling two odd numbers?
b) If you toss two coins, can you work out the probability of getting at least one head?
c) There's a 20% chance that you forgot to take the washing in, and a 50% chance of rain today. What's the probability that your clothes will be soaked?
d) The history teacher gives spot tests on average once every ten lessons, while the maths teacher gives them on average once every five lessons. You have both history and maths today. What's the chance of getting through the day without a test?

NUMBER TRAINING CHALLENGES

1 Imagine you're looking at five red and two black cards face down on the table. Your friend offers you even money that you can't turn over three red cards. Do you take the bet?

2 At an English summer fair in 2,000, there was a stall offering one throw of six dice for £1. If you threw six sixes, you won a new car. What were your chances of driving away with the prize?

3 A bet on red or black at roulette pays even money: you win one chip for a successful bet, and lose one for an unsuccessful bet. The zero is green (so all red/black bets lose on zero), while the other numbers are divided evenly between red and black, 18 each. What's the expected return to £1 bet on red?

4 Can you decipher and continue the following sequences?

   a) 15, 2, 13, 5, 11, 8, __ __ __ (Hint: there are really two sequences in one here.)
   b) 10, 11, 12, 14, 17, 22, 30, 43 __ __ __ (Hint: find the link with a very famous number sequence.)
   c) 26 15 20 20 6 6 19 19 __ __ __ (Hint: think *letters* as well as numbers.)

5 In Blackjack, when the dealer is showing an ace, it's possible for the player to take out 'insurance' against the dealer. If the dealer's second card has a value of ten (i.e. it's a ten, jack, queen or king) then the insurance bet pays 2 to 1. Otherwise the insurance bet loses. Assuming that the game is played with an infinite number of decks (so that cards already played don't affect the odds) what are the odds of a dealer blackjack? And can you calculate the expected return on an insurance bet?

6 Now imagine there's just one deck of cards. The players hands show 9,8 and 4,6,8, and the dealer has an ace. What's the probability of a dealer blackjack in this case? Is insurance a good bet?

7 See how quickly you can slot the missing numbers into this magic square.

9			
4	17		
	1	8	
		15	2

8 There are three buttons, each white on one side and black on the other. Your colleague is offering to pay odds of 2 to 1 if you can throw them in the air and make them land with the same colour showing on all of them. Should you accept the bet?

9 How confident do you feel tackling this mixed set of mental maths questions?

a) 275×200 b) $1,382 - 768$ c) $494 \div 19$ d) $35.89 + 102.55$

10 The barman has taken two kings, two queens and two jacks from a deck. He asks you to take two cards from this set at random, and offers you an even money bet that at least one of your cards will be a queen. Should you take the bet?

8

The formula for success

In this chapter you will learn:
- *that algebra matches the way you think*
- *why variables revolutionize your whole approach to maths*
- *strategies for exploring equations and formulae*
- *how everyday algebra can strengthen vital thinking skills.*

Algebra: letters and numbers, equation-solving, functions, formulae... It's an area of maths that strikes fear into many people's hearts. When you first meet it in school, algebra looks and feels very different from everything that's come before, and it certainly represents a significant change in thinking about numbers, challenging your ideas about what maths is *for*. In the context of this book it provides another excellent opportunity to stretch your brain power in new directions; but the important thing to realize is that algebraic thinking actually comes very naturally. Algebra models what your mind is already doing instinctively.

If your friend told you they were thinking of a number, and that if they divide their number by two they get six, you'd automatically use algebra to tell them that their starting number was 12. 'Half of something is six; so the something must be double six, which is 12.'

Maths just gives us a way to write out this thought process in shorthand:

> *their number / 2 = 6*
> *therefore*
> *their number = 6 × 2 = 12*

You'd also be setting up a rule, a *formula* for solving that sort of question – whatever values were involved: 'Half of their number is the number they tell me; so their number must be double the number they tell me.' In mathematical shorthand this is just

their number / 2 = the number they tell me
therefore
their number = 2 × the number they tell me

It gets quite hard to keep writing 'their number' and 'the number they tell me', so mathematicians tend to give things much shorter names. For example, I could call their missing number n, and the number they tell me a (n for 'number' and a for 'answer'). In this case the equations are written more simply as

$n/2 = a$
therefore
$n = 2 \times a.$

Now whatever a is, we can just substitute its value into the formula, and out pops n – every single time.

When you compare the price of phone networks, negotiate your pay and benefits or calculate the paint you'll need to decorate the living room, you use algebra. You're still finding solutions to the questions you face, but algebra takes your number-thinking a step further.

Arithmetic is about getting fixed answers, but algebra is about defining relationships, giving us new ways to investigate possibilities and to match numbers to changing situations. It requires a delicate blend of logical and creative thinking. You need to pay close attention to details, maintain strong concentration and use your memory to the full. In return, as well as exercising all these key skills, you improve your ability to recognize and analyse patterns and to formulate general rules.

Authors' insight

To cope with algebra you need to have a sound knowledge of the key rules about numbers, an awareness of the relationships between them, and an interest in the way the number system works in general, rather than a fixation on specific answers. It also stretches your brain. It requires excellent reasoning, balanced thinking, strong memory and a high level of concentration. Learn or recap a few key ideas about algebra and you can start finding opportunities to use it every day, boosting many key aspects of your overall brain-training.

So many real-life situations can be explored with algebra. If your company gave its employees a Christmas bonus, you'd use algebra to work out your own December pay – but you'd also be able to describe *everyone's* pay.

December pay (let's call it d) is normal pay (call it n) plus Christmas bonus (call it b):

$$d = n + b$$

You can add together these quantities even though you don't know what they are yet. You're setting up a rule which will give you d whenever you know n and b.

Let's say the bonus is fixed at £150 for everyone.

For everyone, $d = n + 150$

If the boss left it to you to work out how generous he was being, you could look at your pay slip and use a bit of instinctive algebra: 'The bonus must be my December pay minus my normal pay.'

$$b = d - n$$

If you were told what the bonus was, but couldn't remember what you normally got paid...

$$n = d - b$$

If the company decided to organize the bonuses a bit differently this year and give everyone 10% on top of their normal pay:

$$d = n + \frac{10}{100} \times n$$

... and, once again, you'd have a rule for calculating *everyone's* December pay. When the values change, the answer changes, and the question can be investigated from different angles depending on the bits you know.

So algebra is about generalizing rules and thinking flexibly. There's evidence of this kind of approach in ancient Babylon – although the Babylonians solved problems by using algorithms, relying on finite, step-by-step procedures. In Egypt, Greece and China they found the laws of geometry helpful to go beyond specific problems and generalize formulae. Greek mathematician Diophantus used a wide repertoire of techniques to solve equations, described in detail in his series of books called *Arithmetica*, and he's often referred to as 'the father of algebra'. But it was the medieval Muslim mathematician al-Khwarizmi who was the first to present organized methods that worked for other problems: to generalize his rules. Perhaps the paternity of algebra should rightfully be traced to him.

Names in numbers: Al-Khwarizmi

Al-Khwarizmi founded the discipline of *al-jabr*, giving us the word algebra itself, while his name is also enshrined in the word 'algorithm'. He introduced the key ideas of reduction and balancing, which you'll be using to continue your mathematical brain-training in this chapter. His version of algebra was also much more generalized, capable of going beyond a series of fixed problems to find ways of defining the changeable scenarios we meet in everyday life. He wanted to establish mathematical *laws*, and his system provides us all with the tools to do this. We can establish 'mini laws' about the particular situations we face, as well as exploring bigger issues that affect all of us. And Al-Khwarizmi was also fascinated by the study of equations for their own sake. His passion matches the spirit of this chapter, which is about the thinking skills involved in algebra, and the wider benefits they can bring.

Algebra is useful...

... because:

It allows the general formulation of arithmetical laws. Earlier in the book we made use of the fact that $2 + 3$ is the same as $3 + 2$. We said that for *any* two numbers it didn't matter in which order you added them. To write this as a mathematical law we would say that $a + b = b + a$, for all a and b. By replacing a particular number with a symbol which can represent *any* number we can deal with *all* numbers at the same time. One of the most important laws in arithmetic is known as the **distributive law**. It says that $a \times (b + c) = a \times b + a \times c$, for all a, b and c. We use this law all the time without realizing it. For example, when we calculate 4×14 as $4 \times 10 + 4 \times 4 = 40 + 16 = 56$, we're using the distributive law.

It allows us to think about unknown numbers, to put them into equations, and to find ways of solving them. Maya is twice as old as she was four years ago. How old is she now? Giving a label to her unknown age enables us to write down equations representing the information we're given.

If we call her age a, then four years ago her age was $a - 4$. So the information we've got says that $a = 2 \times (a - 4)$. We can simplify this (using the distributive law) to $a = 2 \times a - 8$. So a must be equal to 8.

It allows us to define relationships and to see them in action. It's something you've been doing throughout this book. You already know that if the radius of a circle is R, then its area (call it A) is πR^2 ($\pi \times R \times R$). The formula $A = \pi R^2$ defines the relationship between radius and area for *any* circle. Stick in the radius, out pops the area. Mathematicians often describe this sort of relationship by saying that the area is a *function* of the radius. Similarly the amount of tax you pay is a function of your income. Here the function is described not by a simple formula, but by a complicated set of government rules; but, in the end, if you know your income and the set of rules, you can work out your tax bill. Crucially, the rules tell you how to work out the tax for *any* income.

Algebraic thinking may be instinctive, but simple questions can quickly become complex – and solving them requires more systematic support. The attention to detail and clear logic involved are vital aspects of number training.

'Can you work out my house number? When I multiply it by four and subtract two, the answer is the same as if I'd multiplied it by three and added three.'

With this version of the guess-my-number question, your natural problem-solving tactics would probably match many of the key principles of algebra – with a fair bit of trial-and-error mixed in. You might get lucky and find the number that works, but your approach would be made much more effective by having some simple steps to follow.

The first step is to give the number you're trying to find a label. Let's call it x (for some reason this is a popular choice among mathematicians).

The second step is to write down the information you've got, using the label x in place of the unknown number. In this case:

$$4x - 2 = 3x + 3.$$

The final step is to manipulate this information in order to find the unknown x.

There's a logical approach to manipulating the information, delivering a definitive answer quickly. It relies on the sort of balanced thinking you explored in earlier chapters: 'doing the same to both sides'. You focus on details but also see the whole picture and use all the available information to help you.

You know instinctively that you want to be able to say '$x =$ something', so you need to have x on one side of the equals sign and the answer on the other.

If you add two to the left side, that leaves you with $4x$, and the balance of the equation is maintained by doing the same thing to the right, adding two:

$$4x = 3x + 5.$$

Algebra can give you a great feeling of satisfaction as you see the question simplifying before your eyes and realize you're closing in on the answer. There are four lots of x on the left side now and three lots on the right. We need to collect all the xs together on the same side so subtract three of them from the right, and make sure you do the same on the left:

$$x = 5$$

You've found the definitive answer. The unknown number is now known. In this case, x – the starting number – was 5.

These same three steps – giving the unknowns a label, writing down the information in terms of this label, and manipulating the resulting equation to find the unknown – are used to solve problems in maths (and engineering, physics, theoretical chemistry...) every day. From simple brainteasers to problems about climate change and rocket science the process is the same.

Extracting information

Often the focus of algebra is manipulating equations containing unknown quantities. While this is certainly important, and we'll come to some strategies for it shortly, at least as important is turning the information you're given into an equation in the first place (mathematicians call this 'modelling'). Suppose you hear that Amy is twice as old now as Ben was when Amy was as old as Ben is now.

That's quite a complicated sentence to say, and it (deliberately) obscures the information it contains. Let's label their ages A_{now}, B_{now}, A_{then}, B_{then}. Then you're told that

$$A_{\text{now}} = 2 \times B_{\text{then}} \text{ and}$$

$$A_{\text{then}} = B_{\text{now}}.$$

We also know that Amy ages at the same rate as Ben: $A_{\text{now}} - A_{\text{then}} = B_{\text{now}} - B_{\text{then}}$.

Have a go at extracting the following information. Don't try to solve the equations yet, just see if you can turn the information in words into equations.

Question 1: The sum of my two children's ages is 18, while the product is 80. How old are they?

Question 2: In this family, every boy has the same number of brothers as sisters, but every girl has twice as many brothers as sisters. How many boys and girls are there?

Question 3: Three apples and four oranges cost 41p, while four apples and three oranges cost 36p. What's the price of an apple?

Question 4: Albert, Bertie and Cuthbert were going to split the bill for dinner. But if they'd done so, Albert would have paid 73p too little, while Bertie would have paid 37p too much. So they abandoned that idea and each paid for their own meal. Albert's was £10. How much were the other two?

Rules

Algebra has its own clear rules, based on the logical framework of our number system.

An equation can be manipulated in a variety of ways to do different things. Numbers and letters can be shuffled around on either side of the equals sign – as long as you follow the rules.

- Any quantity can be added to both sides.
- Any quantity can be subtracted from both sides.
- Any quantity can be multiplied to both sides.
- Any quantity can divide both sides (apart from zero).
- Any function can be applied to both sides.

To start strengthening your logical approach and keen eye for detail, have a go with the following equations. Examine each one carefully and then decide which rules will help you to answer the questions underneath.

Question 5:

$x - 4 = 6$

What is $2x$?

Question 6:

$5x = 25$

What is $x + 3$?

Question 7:

$3x + 2 = 11$

Find x.

Question 8:

$6x - 3 = 2x + 9$

Find x.

Question 9:

$x + y = 9$.

What is x?

Mastering algebra involves developing a range of equation-handling tactics. There are decisions to be made about the order in which to carry them out and different ways in which they can be combined, so algebra provides an excellent workout for your creative thinking too.

Some of the key strategies are ...

SIMPLIFYING

Simplification usually involves multiplying out any brackets (using the distributive law) and then combining any terms which can be combined. For example:

$2(3x - 4) + 3(x + 6) = 6x - 8 + 3x + 18 = 9x + 10$.

Question 10: Simplify $8(x - 1) - 3(x + 5) + 2(1 - x)$.

REARRANGING

Rearranging usually means swapping terms to the other side of an equation, so that the term you're focusing on is on its own. An earlier example about Christmas bonuses involved rearranging the equation $d = n + b$. This is the appropriate form if we know n and b and want to calculate d. Then we supposed that we know d and n and wanted to calculate the bonus b. So we rearranged by subtracting n from both sides (and swapping the left- and right-hand sides) to give $b = d - n$. And when we assumed that we knew d and b and wanted to calculate n, we rearranged by subtracting b from both sides to give $n = d - b$.

Question 11: Rearrange the equation $D = S \times T$ (distance is speed multiplied by time) to find expressions for the speed S and the time T in terms of the other two quantities.

GATHERING

When you're solving an equation for x (say), and x appears in more than one place, you need to collect all those terms together if possible. For example, in the equation

$$x = 3x - 2$$

in order to know what x is you need to know what $3x$ is: but how can you know what $3x$ is if you don't know x? It seems you're in an unending loop. The way out is to collect all the xs on one side of the equation. Subtracting x from both sides gives

$$0 = 2x - 2.$$

Adding 2 to both sides gives $2x = 2$. Finally dividing both sides by two gives $x = 1$.

Question 12: Gather similar terms in this equation: $2x + 10 = 6x - 6$.

SUBSTITUTING

There are times when you're faced with more than one equation and more than one unknown. When that happens, if you can solve for one of the unknowns then you can substitute that value wherever the unknown appears, allowing you to solve for the other unknowns. For example, suppose you know that

$$2x + y = 10 \qquad x + 2y = 11$$

You can rearrange the first equation to find that $y = 10 - 2x$. Then you can substitute this value for y into the second equation to give

$$x + 2(10 - 2x) = 11,$$

which you can solve to find $x = 3$. Then you can substitute this into your solution for y to find that $y = 4$.

Question 13: See if you can combine these two equations to get a single equation for x:

$$4x + 2y = 10$$
$$3x + 4y = 15$$

VARIABLE THINKING

So algebra requires a good level of mental flexibility along with the ability to follow clear rules. You also need to be open to new concepts in calculation. As well as working with fixed amounts, *variables* now offer you some exciting possibilities.

Most young children could tell you that seeing eight legs in a field would equate to two cows. If, a few minutes later, the number of legs had gone down to four, they'd be able to readjust their assessment of the situation and explain that there must be only one cow now. They'd be using a simple but very effective formula: the number of cows equals the number of legs divided by four. However many legs they saw, this formula would tell them the number of cows in a single step.

But children need to have a fairly well-developed mathematical mind to understand this thought process as a variable formula and to see its simple brilliance. They're used to using several strategies to solve different sorts of question, but this is something rather different: a solution to every version of this one situation. The answer to the calculation is nowhere near as important as the calculation itself, which will keep working however the scenario changes.

This is how algebra highlights relationships and uses them to take a calculation as far as necessary. The relationship between cows and their number of legs is 1:4. In the following table, describing evolving generations of a species of Lego animal, there's a clear relationship between the animal's number in the sequence and the number of bricks in each of its legs. 'Animal one' has two cubes in its leg, 'animal two' has three ... and so on, presumably; so we can establish a rule that $l = n + 1$. Whatever number we slot into n, we can calculate the number of cubes in its legs, l.

Lego animal number (n)	Bricks in its leg (l)	Bricks in its body (b)
1	2	4
2	3	6
3	4	8
10	$l = n + 1 = 11$	
1000	1001	

Question 14: There's also a clear pattern in the growth of its body; but how do you turn that into a formula so that you don't have to work through the sequence to consider animal 10 or animal 1,000?

Algebra applied

Your creative thinking skills will help you to apply algebra to a range of real-life situations. For example, in the UK in 2009/10 the income-tax free personal allowance was £6,475. After that, the next £37,400 was taxed at the basic rate of 20%. If your taxable income (call it I) was more than £6,475 but less than £43,875, the tax you'd pay (call it T) could be calculated as

$$T = 0.2 (I - 6,475).$$

The amount of money you were left with was

$$I - T = I - 0.2 (I - 6,475) = I - 0.2I + 1,295 = 0.8I + 1,295$$

Or suppose you've got a business selling widgets. You buy a widget at £2 and sell it at £4. You have fixed costs of £10,000 per year. If you sell N widgets a year, what's your profit? How many widgets do you have to sell to break even?

Since the profit per widget is £2, your total profit is $2N - 10,000$ pounds. You break even if this is exactly zero. Then $2N = 10,000$, so that $N = 5,000$. More generally, if the cost price is C, the sale price is S, and the fixed cost is F ... for the profit P you can write:

$$P = N (S - C) - F$$

This general formula lets you answer lots of different questions about the business. For example, suppose you expect to sell only 3,000 widgets. How much do you have to sell them for to make a profit of £2,000? This time N, C, P and F are known but S is unknown. Substituting the values you know gives

$$2{,}000 = 3{,}000(S - 2) - 10{,}000$$

Simplifying and rearranging gives $S = 6$ pounds.

Question 15: If five workers can make 20 widgets in two hours …

a) how many workers will it take to make 14 widgets in one hour?
b) how many hours will it take eight workers to make 12 widgets?
c) how many widgets could three workers make in five hours?
   (Hint: find an equation relating the rate of widget production R (in widgets per hour per worker) to the number of hours, widgets and workers, then do some rearranging to find the quantity you need.)

ALGEBRA BOOSTS YOUR MEMORY

Use the two equations below to practise holding information in front of your 'mind's eye'. Spend a few seconds focusing on the details on the page, then look away and try to describe what you saw from memory.

$$z = \frac{1}{y - \sin(x)}$$

$$F = \frac{Gm_1 m_2}{d^2}$$

Authors' insight

Thinking of objects or people with the appropriate letters, and turning equations into stories, may help you to keep the key information in your memory. You can also visualize equations painted in different colours, the symbols animated or decorated to strengthen their imprint on your mind.

For example, $E = mc^2$

If you were worried about forgetting this famous equation, you might picture Elvis (E) making a sandwich ($=$) out of mayonnaise (m) and cheese (c) and cutting it into a perfect square (^{2}).

Or, to remember $n \times (c + 2)$ …

… how about visualizing your friend Nick (n) blowing a kiss ($\times$) to his cat (c) while it sits in its basket – the brackets, ( ) – with two of its kittens ($+2$)…

Don't worry if your imagery doesn't have anything to do with the real meaning of the maths. In fact, the more surreal and surprising it is, the more memorable it's likely to be. Pick out key details within the information you want to learn and create vivid reminders that will help you reconstruct the rest of it from memory.

Try it out with the next two challenges. Give yourself a minute to study the equations. Look carefully at the letters, numbers and symbols; close your eyes and picture what you saw; use images, stories and anything else that might help you to remember the details; then see how well you get on answering the questions from memory.

Question 16:

$$\binom{n}{k} = \frac{n!}{k!(n-k)!}$$

a) How many times did the letter k appear?
b) How many sets of brackets were there?
c) Can you remember all eight of the characters underneath the line of the fraction?

Question 17:

$$a = \frac{5(4v+3)}{v^2+1} \qquad V = \frac{4}{3}\pi r^3$$

a) Fill in the missing number: $5(4v+ \ldots)$
b) Which number is above a 3?
c) What's on the bottom of the first fraction?

ALGEBRA BOOSTS VISUALIZATION

Do some more mental exercise with the next set of equations. Keep them in front of you as you carry out any of the allowable 'moves' that will get you a value for x. Animate and exaggerate the process in your mind. You can 'extend' your mind by using your hands to mime certain moves, or by imagining the components of the equation rearranging themselves around the room you're sitting in.

Question 18:

$$7x + 5 = 3x - 25$$

Question 19:

$$5x - (3x - 1) = x - 4$$

NUMBER TRAINING CHALLENGES

1 Think flexibly about letters and numbers to help you solve the following question. Agatha is exactly four times as old as Bernard. In ten years she will be three times older than him. How old are Agatha and Bernard now?

2 Yesterday I went fishing. I caught a fish which had a length of 30 cm plus half its own length. How long was the fish?

3 How good are you at spotting the flaw in a mathematical argument? This question returns to the problem of zero: in particular, the dilemma of *dividing* by zero. Many maths tricks and fallacies try to do it when you're not looking ... so keep your eyes open as you explore the following cunning bit of algebra.

The argument is simple: $1 = 0$.

Suppose that $x = 0$.

Multiply both sides by $x - 1$ to get

$$x \times (x - 1) = 0 \times (x - 1) = 0,$$

since any number times zero is zero. Now divide both sides by x to get

$$x - 1 = \frac{0}{x} = 0.$$

since zero divided by anything is still zero. Adding one to both sides gives $x = 1$.

But we started by supposing that $x = 0$. So $0 = 1$. Can you explain what's gone wrong?

4 If Amy, who is five years older than Ben, is twice as old now as Ben was when Amy was as old as Ben is now, how old will Amy be when Ben is as old as Amy is now?

5 Imagine a rope around the equator of the Earth, pulled tight on the Earth's surface. If you added just one metre to the length of the rope, and then somehow managed to hold up the rope so that it was the same height off the ground everywhere ... what height would that be?

6 A single scoop ice-cream cone costs £1, and a double scoop cone costs £2. When my friend put down £2 on the counter, the man behind the counter immediately gave him a double-scoop. But when I put down £2, he asked me which sort of cone I wanted. Use visualization and logic to explain why.

7 The environment agency wants to estimate the number of fish in a lake. They catch 100 fish and tag them, then return a week later and catch another 100 fish. They find that five of these fish are tagged: so, what's a good estimate for the number of fish in the lake?

8 It's time for another mixed set of calculation questions. See how quickly you can solve them in your head.

a) $12 + 16 \times 10.5$ b) $8950 \div 5 - 987$ c) $16^2 - 8^3$
d) $747 \div 9 + 2,079$

9 Here's an exercise in creativity. Add five matches to these six matches to make nine.

10 The answer to this question is a five-digit number. If you put the numeral 1 at the beginning, you get a number three times smaller than if you put the numeral 1 at the end of the number.

9

Think like a mathematician

In this chapter you will learn:
- *why mathematicians search for certainty*
- *different ways of establishing proof*
- *the brain-training benefits of pushing logic to the limit*
- *how mathematical thinking can become a competitive sport.*

Mathematicians look for proof. It's central to the way their minds work. The last chapter showed how algebra provides one way of achieving a definite demonstration of an idea. The rules of algebra have themselves been proved, so they can be used to establish other things beyond doubt. But there are other ways of doing it, using logic, careful reasoning, contradiction... and it's good for you to investigate exactly what mathematicians do as they try to search for certainty.

As well as exercising some important areas of your maths mind, it's a great way of stretching a wide range of thinking skills. You can add a rich new dimension to your memos, meetings, presentations – even your arguments!

A funny way of looking at it

An engineer, a physicist, and a mathematician are travelling by train through the countryside when they see a field full of brown cows. 'Oh,' says the engineer, 'the cows round here are brown.'

'You can't say that,' says the physicist, 'you're assuming too much. All you can say is that the cows in that field are brown.'

'Not true,' says the mathematician. 'All you can say is that at least one side of each cow in that field is brown.'

'Nothing's certain'? Number training puts everything under scrutiny; but, in the end, it might just let you look at the world in a slightly more comfortable way.

And that's exactly how careful mathematicians have to be with their thinking: stating all that they know or assume to be true at the beginning, then seeing what they can derive from it – without making any more assumptions along the way.

Different sorts of proof

Mathematical proof comes in many different forms. Sometimes you can demonstrate directly that a particular result is true. It's also possible to flex your brain in the opposite direction and achieve 'proof by contradiction'. You prove that a particular statement is true by first assuming that the *opposite* is true; then, using the rules of mathematical logic, you follow the consequences of your initial assumption. If somewhere along the line you find yourself at a contradiction, then you know that your initial assumption must be wrong – so the opposite must be true.

Authors' insight

Proof by contradiction is also known by the Latin phrase *reductio ad absurdum*. If the result of following a logical argument leads to an absurd conclusion, then the initial premise must be false. We often do this in everyday life. 'Okay, so you're just going to hand that homework in unfinished, are you? And your teacher's going to be delighted, and understand that you had better things to do all weekend? No, I didn't think so...' We even have colloquial expressions based on it: 'If that's true, then I'm a monkey's uncle'...

Here's what that kind of thinking looks like when a mathematician does it. Look out for the weapons you can borrow for your own argumentative armoury!

Visualize a chessboard and a set of dominoes, each of which covers two squares on the board. Is it possible to cover the whole board of 64 squares with 32 dominoes?

A quick bit of mental manipulation should tell you that the answer is *yes*. In fact there are lots of ways that the dominoes can be arranged to accomplish this.

But what if you remove two squares: the opposite corners of the board?

Exercise your visualization skills by creating that new board in your mind's eye, seeing it from different angles. Make sure you can pick out the stark black and white markings: they might be important details... Now, focus on the question that's been set. Two squares have gone, so you can have one less domino; and is it possible to cover the remaining 62 squares with 31 dominoes?

Authors' insight

In practical tasks, and when you're bending your brain around particularly tricky thinking problems, trial and error is often the best place to start. In a question like 'does multiplying odd numbers ever give an even answer?' it would be sensible to try a few numbers in your head first. '$5 \times 7 = 35$, odd; $13 \times 3 = 39$, odd as well...' So the likelihood is that the answer is *no*, pushing you to pursue the truth in that direction.

So how could you prove that the chessboard challenge is impossible? You could easily build a paper model and try it out. But even with several examples of failure, it could be that you just haven't found the right arrangement of dominoes yet. The fact that *you* can't do it is not enough to prove that *it can't be done*.

The best approach would be to combine two key number-training skills, visualization and logic, to achieve a watertight proof by contradiction.

Think of the pattern of black and white squares on a chessboard, and then imagine a domino covering two squares. Because of the checked pattern, any two adjacent squares are opposite colours, so the domino must cover one black square and one white square. The two squares removed from the board were both the same colour, so the remaining squares must be 32 of one colour and 30 of the other.

Now, if you start by assuming that a covering of the chessboard with 31 dominoes does exist, those dominoes must cover 31 black squares and 31 white squares – so there's the contradiction. It's as simple as that. You can make the confident conclusion that no such covering can possibly exist.

Proof by contradiction is a very powerful mathematical tool, but it's often misunderstood. There are many mathematical theorems like the one above which state that such-and-such can't be done. A common misconception is that, although no one's found it yet, there might still be a way, if we just keep looking. There's an army of amateur mathematicians seeking fame and fortune by trying to find ways of doing things which have been *proved* impossible. It's probably very good brain training – but sometimes you just need to know when to stop!

Names in numbers: Lewis Carroll

Lewis Carroll, born Charles Lutwidge Dodgson, is most famous as the author of *Alice's Adventures in Wonderland*, but he was also a leading Oxford University maths professor with an incredible appetite for a challenge. As well as pushing his own maths mind to devise systems for, among other things, sorting electoral battles, organizing tennis tournaments and cracking complex codes, he wrote a number of books packed with entertaining and challenging puzzles. He was keen to show the magic of maths and to demonstrate the pleasures and practical benefits attached to his brand of brain training. But perhaps it's the *Alice* books themselves that are his richest source of maths challenges, stretching the thinking of readers young and old.

They represent a wonderful combination of logic and creativity, exploring challenging aspects of mathematical thinking in some delightful and ingenious ways.

Here are just a few of the intriguing issues Lewis Carroll tackles. See what they do for *your* brain.

At The Pool of Tears, Alice gets very muddled with multiplication. 'Let me see: four times five is twelve, and four times six is thirteen, and four times seven is – oh dear! I shall never get to twenty at that rate!' But is she really exploring what happens to numbers in different bases and using different positional systems? In base 18 notation, $4 \times 5 = 12$ (two in the 'ones' column, one in the 'eighteens'). $4 \times 6 = 13$ if you're using base 21 notation. And if you continue this sequence, going on three more bases to 24... 4×7 can indeed be represented as 14.

Question 1: Is Alice right? If she keeps going with this sequence, will she 'never get to twenty'?

At the 'Mad Tea Party', the March Hare, Mad Hatter and Dormouse get into a complex conversation that seems to be about mathematical logic and inverse relationships. '*Why, you might just as well say that "I see what I eat" is the same thing as "I eat what I see"!*' Logic is also stretched to breaking point in Chapter 5 when the Pigeon explains confidently that a little girl must be a kind of serpent, because both little girls and serpents eat eggs.

Question 2: What would you say to prove the Pigeon wrong?

And when the Cheshire Cat keeps fading until all that's left is its grin, Alice comments that she's seen a cat without a grin, but never a grin without a cat. This sort of abstract thinking was big news in maths at the time – not entirely to Lewis Carroll's liking – and it certainly opens up some brain-bending ideas.

You might have two or three girls or books or cats, and you could quite easily consider those physical things themselves, separate from their numbers. But what happens when you try it the other way, thinking just of the 'two' or 'three', no longer connected to their 'things'? If physical objects can exist without numbers, what happens to numbers when they get separated from their objects, like grins separated from cats…?

When you start challenging your maths mind it can lead you in some very unusual directions. Why not re-read some of Lewis Carroll's books and see what they do to your brain the second time around!

Names in numbers: Priyanshi Somani

At just 12 years old, Priyanshi Somani was the youngest participant of the Mental Calculation World Cup in 2010 – and yet she won the overall title. Her phenomenal feats included multiplying two eight-digit numbers, adding ten ten-digit numbers, and extracting square roots from numbers of six digits. American psychologist Michael O'Boyle has carried out MRI scans during competitions like this. He's been able to show that leading calculators experience surges in blood flow to key brain areas. Maths prodigies can achieve up to seven times faster blood flow to parts of their brain responsible for mathematical thinking.

Prizefighters

Maths can be a wonderfully competitive sport. As well as struggling to find ways of understanding the world and explaining our experiences of it, mathematicians have often found time to battle against each other. A competitive spirit seems to be a very important aspect of maths thinking. It pushes mathematicians to find better ways to use their brains, ensuring that they're always searching for new perspectives and clearer insights as they challenge the ideas of others.

The history of maths is full of heated arguments and competing theories. One particular showdown in sixteenth century Italy, about how to solve complex equations, led to two leading mathematicians, Tartaglia and Fiore, facing off in a head-to-head trial of algebraic agility.

'Fermat's Last Theorem' sparked a global battle as mathematicians vied to provide proof for a deceptively simple bit of number theory. Frenchman Pierre de Fermat claimed to have it sorted back in 1637, but it was 358 years before British mathematician Andrew Wiles supplied conclusive proof and claimed the $50,000 prize.

There are many other contests around the world at which number-trained brains can shine. And if you're interested in earning fame and fortune with your reinvigorated thinking skills, there are plenty of maths prizes on offer.

If you're under 40 there's the prestigious Fields Medal, honouring Canadian mathematician John Charles Fields and awarded to leading maths minds every four years, with a prize of around $15,000. Every year the king of Norway presents the Abel prize, after legendary mathematician Niels Henrik Abel, which could earn you a share of around a million dollars. And then there are the Clay Millennium Prizes: seven million dollars offered for solving seven of the most difficult problems in existence at the turn of the millennium. The fund has just dropped to six, because the Poincaré Conjecture has recently been proved; but you should have time to try your luck with the others, if you're quick...

NUMBER TRAINING CHALLENGES

1   William Briggs features the following intriguing puzzle in his book *Ants, Bikes and Clocks*. Picture a jigsaw containing 1,000 pieces. A section is a set of pieces (even just one piece) which are already connected. A move means joining two sections. What is the smallest number of moves required to complete the jigsaw?

2   Put your logical thinking to the test. In a group, half of the people are women, and half of the people are coffee drinkers. Does it follow that ½ × ½ = ¼ of the people are female coffee drinkers? And are half of the men coffee drinkers?

3   What's the easiest method of adding all the numbers from one to 100?

4   How quickly and accurately can you solve the following percentage problems?

   a) 20% of 55   b) 16% of 75   c) 17.5% of 280   d) 8% of 250

5   Imagine you've managed to collect three discount coupons for a local restaurant. One is for 25%, one for 35% and one for 40%. There's nothing in the smallprint that says you can't combine offers, so you decide to visit the restaurant and claim your free meal – because 25% + 35% + 40% = 100% discount. The restaurant manager says he's happy to honour each of your vouchers, and you can apply them all to the same bill, but there will still be some money to pay. What does he mean, and how much will you owe?

6   117 players enter a tennis tournament. In each round, names are drawn out of a hat in pairs until all players are paired up. These pairings determine the matches played in that round. The losing players are eliminated, while the winners go through to the next round. If there's an odd number of players in a round then the final player drawn is given a bye. So, there are 58 matches in the first round, one player gets a bye, and there are 59 players in the second round. How many matches will have to be played before a winner is crowned?

7   The tail of a fish is as long as its head and a quarter of its body. The body is three quarters of the total length. The head is four inches long. How long is the fish?

8   Focus on the facts of this question very carefully. There's a town where 3/10 of the men and 2/5 of the women are married. Assuming that all married couples live in the town itself, and that each person has only one spouse, what percentage of the townspeople are single men?

9   Have you got the memory skills of a mathematician? Use any of the tricks explained in Chapter 6 to recall the third, fifth and seventh decimal places of pi.

10 Is it true that, on average, people in the UK have fewer than two legs?

10

Big maths, big challenges

In this chapter you will learn:
- *techniques for coping with very big and very small numbers*
- *more about accurate estimating*
- *how to challenge your maths mind with ideas about infinity*
- *advice for keeping your number-training going.*

… and then there's the companion test to the one you took at the beginning, to let you see whether our particular brand of brain training is working for you.

This chapter is about how big (and small) maths can be, and where it can take your thinking. As well as the questions at the end, there are features throughout to gauge your ability and confidence to deal with some very challenging concepts. We've included examples of the fun and fascinating side of maths to keep you going, even when the going gets tough, and we hope this chapter will inspire you to continue expanding your maths mind: finding brain-training opportunities in daily life but also pushing yourself to tackle some of the biggest questions of all.

Big and small numbers

Numbers with three or four digits are easy to read, but any longer than that and it's tricky to see the true value. The 'start' is sufficiently far from the 'end' for us to lose our place – unless we insert a signpost of some sort. In the UK this is done by inserting a comma after every three digits, counting from the units column 'forwards'. So 10345 becomes 10,345 and we can quickly see that the number is 10 thousand and something. Once we get above six digits we insert another comma, so that 1234567 becomes 1,234,567 and we can see immediately that the number is 1 million and something. In these days of spiralling national debt and global populations, we occasionally come across even larger numbers. 5656123675 becomes 5,656,123,675: 5 billion and something.

After this it gets tricky again. Even with the commas as signposts it's difficult to count the groups of three digits, and we start to lose track again – and to run out of words.

In everyday situations we rarely meet numbers in the trillions, but in the scientific world they're not uncommon. So, scientists have a shorthand way for writing such large numbers (sometimes called *scientific notation*). It's also true that if a number is in the billions you don't really care about its exact value: often getting it to the nearest million will be enough.

SCIENTIFIC NOTATION

In scientific notation you count the number of powers of ten in a number. And to do that you just keep moving the digits to the right (which corresponds to dividing by ten) and multiplying by ten (so that the number is unchanged), until you have a number between one and ten. So:

$$10,345 = 1034.5 \times 10 = 103.45 \times 10^2 = 10.345 \times 10^3 = 1.0345 \times 10^4.$$

As you saw in Chapter 3, multiplying and dividing by powers of ten is a good way to practise focused visualization, moving sets of digits left or right across the place value columns while keeping the decimal point firmly fixed.

Question 1: Focus on the details, follow the logic and find the scientific notation for the following numbers:

a) 1,234,567   b) 5,656,123,676   c) 93,790,003,984.833

And when you've done that... spend a moment contemplating just how big these numbers are. Remember, 1×10^9 is a 1 followed by 9 zeros.

A similar approach works with very small numbers (and here you don't even have the commas to help you!). For small numbers, even 0.01 becomes hard to identify quickly. To write these numbers in scientific notation, keep moving the digits one place to the left while dividing by ten until you get a number between one and ten.

$$0.134 = \frac{1.34}{10} = 1.34 \times 10^{-1}.$$

$$0.003456 = \frac{0.03456}{10} = \frac{0.3456}{10^2} = \frac{3.456}{10^3} = 3.465 \times 10^{-3}.$$

Question 2: See how quickly you can convert these small numbers into scientific notation. Don't write anything down or even touch the numbers on the page. Do it all in your number-trained brain.

a) 0.00039   b) 0.0000607008   c) 0.0000001101001

Authors' insight

The balanced thinking you've developed throughout your number training should help you to spot that dividing by a power of ten corresponds to multiplying it by the *negative* power of ten.

Thinking to scale

When you're dealing with very big or very small numbers, it's particularly important to include estimation in your thought process. It can help to think of it in terms of scaling. For example, when dealing with large numbers, say $1{,}531 \times 19{,}625$, estimation instructs you to be aware of the number of digits expected for the final value.

$1{,}531$ is around $1{,}500$, and $19{,}625$ is around $20{,}000$, so a result of around $20{,}000 \times 1{,}500$ ($30{,}000{,}000$) would be a good estimate for the actual answer ($30{,}045{,}875$). If your answer has too many digits, you know you've made a mistake.

Authors' insight

Experiments have shown that our estimates vary depending on how a question is posed. When volunteers were asked to estimate the answer to $9 \times 8 \times 7 \times 6 \times 5 \times 4 \times 3 \times 2 \times 1$, their average response was 4,200. But when the question was put the other way round, $1 \times 2 \times 3 \ldots \times 9$, the average went down to 500. It seems we start our estimates with an 'anchor' amount, the one that first comes to mind, and adjust up or down from that. In a question like this, the first few numbers influence our anchor, and we're not very good at adjusting sufficiently from that initial guess (although perhaps the flexibility of thought developed through number training will improve that...) Shops will still make use of this principle when they price their goods: £4.99 points our brains more towards £4 than £5, even though it's only a penny away. Charities will continue to suggest high donations – 'You might like to pledge £50, £25, £10, £5' – to fix our 'anchor' amount high and influence our estimation of how much is appropriate to give.

To infinity and beyond

Is your brain ready to cope with the concept of infinity? If you think it is, then you'd better be prepared for more than one...

DIFFERENT TYPES OF INFINITY

If we add something to a set, the set gets bigger: we know that instinctively. But when we're dealing with infinite sets, intuition can lead us astray.

Before we can talk about different types of infinity, we need a way to compare the sizes of two infinite sets of objects.

As always, switch on your visualization. Imagine you want to see which of two boxes contains the most apples. You could count the apples in each box, and compare the two totals; but you only need to know which box has the most, not how many there are in each box, so instead you could simply pair off the apples. If both boxes become empty at the same time then they must have started with the same number of apples. If one box has apples remaining when the other's empty, then that box must have started with more.

You can use this 'pairing up' method to compare the sizes of infinite sets of objects. If you can pair up each object in the first set with one from the second, so that no objects are missed out or left over, then the two sets are said to be the same size.

Suppose that one of the sets is the simplest of all infinite sets: the set of whole numbers 1, 2, 3, ... If each object in a set can be paired up with a whole number, so that no numbers or objects are left out, then the set is said to be *countable*, or *countably infinite*. For sets like that we can list the objects in a sequence, the number paired with 1 listed first, the number paired with 2 second, and on, and on ... This is the 'smallest' type of infinity considered by mathematicians, but it can still produce some surprises.

If you've got a countably infinite set of objects, and you add one more, how many do you have? The set is countable so it can be written as a list, and all you have to do is put the new object at the front of the list. You pair the new object with 1, and whatever used to be paired with 1 now goes with 2... So you still have a countable set. Infinity plus one equals... *infinity*.

This German mathematician visualized infinity in a hotel. His imaginary hotel has an infinite number of rooms, all of them occupied. Although the hotel is full, when a new guest arrives they can be accommodated by asking all the existing guests to each move to the next room, so that the guest in room 1 moves to room 2, the person in room 2 moves to room 3, and so on. This leaves room 1 vacant for the new visitor.

By repeating the process, any finite number of new arrivals can be accommodated. But in fact the hotel is stranger still. Suppose an infinite number of guests arrive. The manager then simply asks each guest to move to the room number which is double their current room number. This leaves all the odd numbered rooms free for the new guests, showing that $\infty + \infty = \infty$.

A BIGGER INFINITY

But are there any sets that are not countable? Is there a bigger infinity? The answer to this question is *yes*. There are more numbers than there are whole numbers: the set of all numbers is not countable.

Challenge your logical thinking by pursuing another proof by contradiction. Suppose the numbers between zero and one were countable. Then they could be listed as a sequence $a_0, a_1, a_2, \ldots$ If you can show that there's a number which isn't in the sequence anywhere, then you'll have found the contradiction.

To construct a number not in the sequence, imagine a number between zero and one which is different from a_0 in the tenths column, different from a_1 in the hundredths column, different from a_2 in the 3rd decimal place… In each case there are nine other digits to choose from, so there are plenty of ways to do this. But the number you've imagined can't be on the list – because it's different from every number that *is* there.

TAKING IT TO THE LIMIT

Push your maths brain to the edge of the universe and back again.

Question 3: How many times can you fold a piece of paper – any piece of paper – in half? The creative answer might be *once*, since after that it would be folded in quarters, eighths and so on, but you know what we mean: folding the paper to halve it, and then halving what's left. Picture yourself doing it, then check the answer at the end of the chapter to test your visualization and estimation skills.

In John D. Barrow's book *100 Essential Things You Didn't Know You Didn't Know*, he imagines cutting a piece of paper in half, first with scissors and then with a laser, halving it 114 times until the remaining piece measures 10^{-33} cm – which takes you beyond the reach of physics. And if you could double the size of an A4 sheet of paper, after 90 doublings it would stretch to the edge of the entire visible universe, 14 billion light years away. So just 204 halvings and doublings take you from the smallest to the largest points of physical reality. Maths really does stretch your thinking skills to the limits.

Big possibilities

When people are fitted with cochlear implants, electronic gadgets which allow them to hear, their brains have to adapt to cope – and they do. A sort of 'rewiring' goes on to allow the user to process sounds created electronically. It doesn't happen instantly, but gradually the changes become apparent and the person gets used to using their brain in a new way.

This book has offered ideas and activities to help you start using your brain better, and maybe to *change* it for the better. Now it's up to you to continue the process. Stay alert to all the opportunities to stretch your core thinking skills. Enjoy the fun and fascination involved in exploring the world with numbers, shapes and mathematical ideas. Apply your improved understanding of maths whenever and wherever you can and look out for the knock-on effects on other aspects of your thinking.

Albert Einstein said his talent lay in being 'merely inquisitive'. His questioning led to phenomenal feats of creative visualization.

The great A. C. Aitken saw interesting numbers everywhere he looked – and used them to carry out his breathtaking mental calculations.

When a colleague observed that his taxi number 1729 was not particularly interesting, Indian mathematician Srinivasa Ramanujan replied that on the contrary, it represented 'the smallest number expressible as the sum of two cubes in two different ways'.

We want you to keep using the specific thinking skills you've learned in this book, to tackle mathematical challenges but also to help in every other part of your life. And we hope you'll simply enjoy the feeling of having a mind in tune with the principles, processes and patterns of numbers and able to cope brilliantly with all the maths it meets.

NUMBER TRAINING
CHALLENGES

1 Imagine you've come to a fork in the road and need to know which is the right way to your destination. The good news is that there are two local men at the roadside, and both of them know the way. The bad news is that one of them always tells the truth, the other one always lies – and you don't know which is which. You've got only one question to put to either of the men. So, what do you say?

2 How quickly can you convert these very big and very small numbers into scientific notation?

a) 5,670,000
b) 4765.4532
c) 0.00000000123
d) 43,543,123,982.25

3 Five pirates are dividing up their treasure – 100 gold coins. There's a clear pecking order among the pirates. The boss is pirate number 1, and the tea-boy is pirate number 5. They also have a very particular method of allocating shares of the treasure. The lowest-ranked pirate proposes a division, and then they hold a vote. If the vote passes by a clear majority, then the division is accepted. If it fails, the proposing pirate is killed. There is then one fewer pirate and it falls to the new lowest ranking pirate to propose a division of the treasure among those remaining. The pirates are greedy – and highly logical. They will always vote for a proposal if they stand to gain more treasure that way. On the other hand, if they gain an equal amount of treasure by voting for or against a proposal they will always vote *against*, killing the proposer. They are pirates, after all...

Imagine you're pirate number 5. Use your number-trained brain to the full to work out the proposal that will keep you alive and win you the biggest possible share of the treasure.

4 A prime number is a number that has exactly two whole-number factors: the number itself, and one. So three is a prime number (only divisible by 3 and 1), and so are 5, 7, 11, 13, 17... Is it true that all prime numbers greater than three are either one less or one more than a multiple of six?

5 When you're writing numbers in words, how far do you have to count before you use the letter A? Be logical, visualize, and focus on the details you see.

6 Look carefully at the matchstick picture below. Can you move four matches to create three squares – and find two solutions?

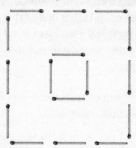

7 Use your focused thinking, concentration and creativity to work out what's special about this large number: 8,549,176,320.

8 When it's read from left to right, which two-digit number is exactly 4½ times smaller than when you read it from right to left?

9 This question exercises your memory and concentration. It works best if you can get someone to read it to you.

Imagine you're driving a bus from the coast to the city. At the first stop, eight people get on board. At the second stop, five get on and three get off. At the next stop, half the passengers get off and six get on. Six people leave the bus at the next stop, but ten get on. A third of the passengers get off at the next stop and seven get on. Then, just one stop from the end of the line, three passengers get off. The question is: what's the name of the driver?

10 Concentrate through all the steps of the following question and find the cleverest ways to get to the final answer.

Start with a million. Divide it by four. Divide the result by five. Divide the result of that by two. Divide the new result by 20. Subtract 50. Divide by three. Divide that result by eight. Subtract one. Divide the result of this by seven. Add two. Divide the result by three. Add two. Divide this result by five. What are you left with?

Test yourself now

Use this final set of challenges to put your number-trained brain through its paces – and to see how it feels now. Although the questions are grouped under the key thinking skills explored in the book, many of them will stretch several 'bits' of your brain. In fact, the ability to use all your maths skills flexibly and creatively may well be the best indication that your training is paying off.

VISUALIZATION

1 Picture the keypad of your mobile phone. Hold this number square in your mind as you answer the following questions.
   a) Find the number in the middle of each side of the square and add all four together.
   b) Add the number above 7 to the number below 6 and multiply the answer by the number below 2.
2 Typed into a calculator, what would the following numbers look like upside down?
   a) 07734
   b) 0.0791
   c) 53177187714
3 If you're facing South West and turn 90 degrees anticlockwise, then 180 degrees, then 270 degrees clockwise, 135 degrees anticlockwise and finally 225 degrees clockwise... which way are you facing now?

4 Spend one minute memorizing the following grid of numbers.

4	3	0	5
2	0	1	7
7	4	3	8
1	6	9	5

Now cover the grid and answer these questions from memory:
   a) What are the digits in the four middle squares?
   b) How many 3s are there?
   c) Which number is above the 8?
   d) What is the product of the four corner digits?

5 Carry out the following five calculations, in order, from memory. Work out the letter values of your answers – but this time, work from the back of the alphabet to the front: $1 = Z$, $2 = Y$, $3 = X$… Then you'll need to rearrange the letters to produce the final answer, and do it all in your head.

a)	26×2	$+229$	-101	$\div 60$	$+19$
b)	105×3	-25	$\div 2$	-58	-75
c)	$126 \div 7$	$\times 4$	$+280$	$\div 22$	-12
d)	17×5	$+297$	-49	$\div 111$	$\times 3$
e)	$1{,}009 + 111$	$\div 2$	$+551$	$\div 11$	-90

6 Give yourself a minute to study the equation below, then cover it up as you answer the questions from memory.

$$f(x) = \sum_{n=0}^{\infty} a_n (x-a)^n.$$

a) How many times does the letter n appear in this equation?
b) Which symbol is above Σ?
c) What's inside the brackets?

EXTENDED MIND

7 You've experimented with several techniques for using your hands to extend your thinking. Now try going further and use the room you're sitting in to help you deal with numbers.

Step 1: Working round the four corners of the room in a clockwise direction, imagine seeing the following four numbers carved into the walls: 7, 16, 11, 34.

Step 2: Cover up Step 1 and check you can still visualize the four numbers in the corners of the room.

Step 3: With the numbers still covered, use the room to help you remember and manipulate the four numbers as you answer the following questions:

a) What's the total of the four numbers?
b) Multiply the first number by the one diagonally opposite it in the room.
c) Subtract the first two numbers from the second two.
d) Imagine standing in the corner marked 16. Taking that as your starting number, add on the number diagonally opposite, then subtract the number to your right – and, whatever you get, multiply it by the number on your left. What's your final answer?

FOCUSED THINKING

8 Examine the following 'proof' that $2 = 1$.

$a = x$ (which is true for some values of a and some values of x)
$a + a = a + x$ (add a to both sides)
$2a = a + x$ (simplifying the previous line)
$2a - 2x = a + x - 2x$ (subtract $2x$ from both sides)
$2(a - x) = a + x - 2x$ (simplifying again)
$2(a - x) = a - x$ (and again)
$2 = 1$ (divide both sides by $(a - x)$

Can you spot the flaw in the argument?

LOGIC

9 Brothers or sisters have I none, but that man's father is my father's son. Who is that man?

10 True or false: if 50% of the group are women, and 30% of the group are mathematicians, then 15% of the group are female mathematicians.

11 Can you explain the very first puzzle in the Introduction of this book?

CREATIVITY

12 You need to take a 5 ft long curtain pole home on the bus, but you know that the driver won't let you on with any item longer than 4 ft in any dimension. What could you use to solve this problem and get your pole home?

13 Henry Dudeney created this famously challenging puzzle – an advancement of one you tried earlier in the book. Can you make 100 by using all the digits from one to nine in order, inserting *exactly* three symbols to get you to the target?

14 Imagine a cherry in a wine glass – depicted by matchsticks and a coin. By moving only two matchsticks, can you get the cherry out of the glass? The cherry can't be trapped underneath the glass, and the glass still needs to look like a glass at the end!

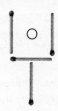

Taking it further

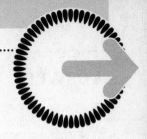

BOOKS

Barrow, J. D., *100 Essential Things You Didn't Know You Didn't Know* (Bodley Head, 2008).

Crilly, T., *50 Mathematical Ideas You Really Need to Know* (Quercus Publishing, 2007).

Acheson, D., *1089 and All That: a Journey into Mathematics* (Oxford University Press, 2002).

Briggs, W., *Ants, Bikes and Clocks: Problem Solving for Undergraduates* (SIAM, 2005).

Buchan, J., *As Easy as Pi* (Michael O'Mara Books, 2009).

vos Savant, M. and Fleischer, L., *Brain Power* (Piatkus, 2009).

Stewart, I., *Math Hysteria* (Oxford University Press, 2004).

Budd, C. J. and Sangwin, C. J., *Mathematics Galore!* (Oxford University Press, 2001).

Potter, L., *Mathematics Minus Fear* (Marion Boyars, 2006).

Staffod, T. and Webb, M., *Mind Hacks* (O'Reilly Media, 2004).

WEBSITES

www.cut-the-knot.org

www.mathsisfun.com

www.numericana.com

www.syvum.com/teasers

....

Answers

Introduction to number training

1 A regular hexagon
2 6
3 4 (but two of them will make all the matches fall out!)
4 1

TEST YOURSELF NOW

1 You need to build a 3D shape: a tetrahedron, with four
   triangular faces.
3 It depends on how you draw the letters... but the best answer is
   probably 16: A B C D E H I K M O T U V W X Y
4 North
6 a) 2 (B) b) 18 (R) c) 1 (A) d) 9 (I) e) 14 (N) = BRAIN
8 a) yes b) yes c) no d) 5
9 Don't be fooled by the clever wording of this famous question.
   The amounts picked out shouldn't add up to £30. In the end, the
   meal only cost £25: and, although they paid £27 altogether, £2
   of the men's money ended up with the waitress, and £27 minus
   £2 is £25.
10 The man in front knows he's wearing a black hat, and here's
   how. The first man cannot have seen two white hats, since
   otherwise he would have known that his own hat was black. So
   the second man knows that at least one of the second and third
   hats is black. If he himself saw a white hat on the third man, he
   would know that his own hat must be black. Because he didn't
   know the colour of his hat, he must have seen a black hat on the
   third man.
11 Place the coin at the top of the L *on top of* the one at the corner,
   so that there are four coins in each line.
12 Add a diagonal line to the second plus sign to turn it into a 4, so
   that the sum reads: 5 + 545 = 550. (Or, just put a diagonal line
   through the equals sign, to mean 'not equals'!)
13 On a clock – two hours after 11 is one o'clock.

Chapter 1

1 a) 37   b) 34   c) 33
2 193
3 a) 470   b) 89200   c) 30.23   d) 438   e) 479   f) 7.833206
   g) 0.0000308   h) 394,304,820
4 a) 1001110   b) 10000001
5 The code-word is DOUBLING.
6 The four answers represent the year this book was first
   published: 2011.

NUMBER TRAINING CHALLENGES

1 4 (because there are four letters in the word 'four').
2 112
3 Altogether, there are 12 faces on the two cubes. Both need to
   have a 1 and a 2, to make 11 and 22; both must also have 0,
   to make 0 to 9 (01, 02, etc.) as well as 10, 20 and 30. That
   leaves just six faces, three on each cube, and seven numbers are
   required, 3 to 9. But 6 will become 9 when it's turned upside
   down: so cube A has the digits 0, 1, 2, 3, 4, 5, and cube B 0, 1, 2,
   6 (which can also be 9), 7, and 8.
4 168
5 The binary codes represent 3, 5, 7 and 9 – so the next number
   in this odd-number sequence is 11: which, in binary notation,
   is 1011.
6 The first ten numbers in ternary code – base three – would be:
   1, 2, 10, 11, 12, 20, 21, 22, 100, 101.
7 a) In binary, the starting positions are 101, 111, 1001. You
      should play first. You need to add or subtract an 8, a 2 and a
      1. From the pile of 9 subtract 7 (which is plus 8, minus 2,
      plus 1).
   b) In binary, these are 111, 1011, 1101. The digit sums are all
      even except for the 1s column, so you need to take one from
      any pile.
   c) This time the binary codes are 110, 1001, 1111. All the digit
      sums are even, so you should play second.
8 The answers are numbers in the Fibonacci sequence: 0, 1, 1, 2, 3,
   5, 8, 13, 21. The next number would be 13 + 21 = 34.

9 On a regular number line, −23 to 49 would be 72. But the answer is actually 71, because there wasn't a 'year zero'.

10 If Amy had 1 or 10, she would have solved the puzzle straight away; but she didn't, so we (and Ben) know that she couldn't have had either of those numbers. If Ben had 1 or 10 he would also have solved the puzzle straight away. Since he knows after Amy's first answer that she doesn't have 1 or 10, he would also have solved it if he had 2 or 9, since then he would know that she must have 3 or 8 respectively. So we know that Ben doesn't have 1, 2, 9 or 10. On hearing this, Amy knows the answer. So she must have a number which is next to 1, 2, 9 or 10. For example, if Amy has 2, she knows that Ben has 3 (since he can't have 1). And if Amy has 3 she knows that Ben has 4 (since he can't have 2). But if Amy has 4, she still wouldn't know whether Ben had 3 or 5. So the four possible solutions are 2 and 3, 3 and 4, 9 and 8, and 8 and 7.

Chapter 2

1 0 + 10, 2 + 8, 4 + 6, 1 + 9, −5 + 15, −4 + 14

2 27 + 73, 41 + 59, 75 + 25, 21 + 79, 28 + 72

3 a) 65 b) 87 c) 572 d) 366

4 a) wrong b) wrong c) right

5 a) 38 b) 35 c) 17

6 None. All the birds will fly away as soon as they hear the gunshot.

7 The completed magic square looks like this.

7	12	1	14
2	13	8	11
16	3	10	5
9	6	15	4

It's called the Chautisa Yantra. Each row, column, diagonal, 2 × 2 sub-square, the corners of each 3 × 3 and 4 × 4 square, the two sets of four symmetrical numbers (1 + 11 + 16 + 6 and 2 + 12 + 15 + 5), and the sum of the middle two entries of the two outer columns and rows ($12 + 1 + 6 + 15$ and $2 + 16 + 11 + 5$), all add up to 34.

8 a) 454   b) 974   c) 2,145
9 a) 21   b) 99   c) 39   d) 35

NUMBER TRAINING CHALLENGES

1 Move one of the lines from the equals sign and combine it with the minus sign to give $101 = 102 - 1$.

2 $12 + 14$, $2 + 24$, $13 + 13$, $-6 + 32$, $-4 + 30$.

3 The solutions are:

$12 + 3 - 4 + 5 + 67 + 8 + 9 = 100$
$123 - 4 - 5 - 6 - 7 + 8 - 9 = 100$
$123 + 4 - 5 + 67 - 89 = 100$
$123 + 45 - 67 + 8 - 9 = 100$
$123 - 45 - 67 + 89 = 100$
$12 - 3 - 4 + 5 - 6 + 7 + 89 = 100$
$12 + 3 + 4 + 5 - 6 - 7 + 89 = 100$
$1 + 23 - 4 + 5 + 6 + 78 - 9 = 100$
$1 + 23 - 4 + 56 + 7 + 8 + 9 = 100$
$1 + 2 + 3 - 4 + 5 + 6 + 78 + 9 = 100$
$-1 + 2 - 3 + 4 + 5 + 6 + 78 + 9 = 100$

4 The first 20 numbers of the Fibonacci Sequence are: 1, 1, 2, 3, 5, 8, 13, 21, 34, 55, 89, 144, 233, 377, 610, 987, 1597, 2584, 4181, 6765

5 a) 62   b) 279   c) 431   d) 69
6 a) 177   b) 411   c) 7,620   d) 32,303
7 There are two possible answers. Your finished square should look like one of these:

9	6	3	16
4	15	10	5
14	1	8	11
7	12	13	2

13	6	3	12
4	11	14	5
10	1	8	15
7	16	9	2

8 a) 9   b) 95   c) 79   d) 1939
9 a) 18   b) 70   c) 89   d) 987
10 a) 5   b) 20   c) 20   d) 19 = TEST

Chapter 3

1 a) right b) wrong c) right d) wrong e) right f) wrong
2 a) 966 b) 3,195 c) 7,953 d) 43,260
3 a) 21 remainder 5 b) 11 remainder 29 c) 24 remainder 16
 d) 12 remainder 30
4 There are 22 factors besides 1 and 360: 2, 3, 4, 5, 6, 8, 9, 10, 12,
 15, 18, 20, 24, 30, 36, 40, 45, 60, 72, 90, 120, 180
5 a) 870,000 b) 232 c) 570 d) 576 e) 960
6 a) −25 b) 79 c) 400 d) 9
7 It takes 111 steps before you get to the number 1.
8 a) 28 b) 64 c) 18 d) 60 e) 54 f) 77 g) 24 h) 56
 i) 27 j) 42 k) 45 l) 32 m) 36 n) 36 o) 48
9 a) 264 b) 4,202 c) 4,796 d) 30,118 e) 1,044,318
10 a) 156 b) 483 c) 592 d) 3,630

NUMBER TRAINING CHALLENGES

1 a) 348 b) 2,240 c) 640 d) 1,584
2 zero
3 a) 2,926 b) 2,535 c) 5,528
4 a) 158 b) 272 c) 492 d) 2,940
5 a) 198 b) 182 c) 726
6 a) 27 b) 23 c) 46
7 She has three girls. Half of them are girls, and the other half are
 also girls.
8 Three cuts. When you cut a link, you can remove the links
 from each side. So first cutting the middle link will give
 you one link, and two chains, each three links long. Then
 cutting each of those in the middle will divide the chain into
 individual links.

 But... if the gardener agrees not to spend his links just yet, you
 could do it with a single cut – to the link three from the end of
 the chain. This would give you a single link, a chain of two and
 a chain of four. On day one you could hand over the one link.
 On day two, you'd ask for that link back and replace it with the
 chain of two. On day three, you'd need to give the single link
 again... and so on until day seven when the gardener had all
 seven links.

9   The creative solution is to cut each of the three pills in half and put the halves into two separate piles. You know that each pile contains two halves of B and half of A. So take a new pill from the A bottle, cut it in half and add a piece to each pile. Now there must be a whole B and whole A pill in each pile. Take one pile today and the other tomorrow.

10 The farmer's clever idea was to borrow a sheep for a while. Sixteen is a much easier number to halve. So the first boy received eight sheep, the second four, the third two, the fourth one… and then the single sheep left was simply returned.

Chapter 4

1   Add a decimal point to give 5.9.

2   a) ¼ = 10/40   b) 3/5 = 12/20   c) 3/20 = 150/1000
    d) 1 ½ = 270/180

3   a) 1.75 = 1 ¾   b) 4/5 = 0.8   c) 33.333 = 100/3 = 33 1/3
    d) 60/80 = 0.75

4   a) 2/5 = 40%   b) 1.8 = 180%   c) 72% = 18/25
    d) 122% = 1 11/50

5   a) 75%   b) 2/17   c) 0.2   d) 12/25

6   a) ¼   b) 0.08   c) 54

7   a) Yes   b) No   c) Yes

8   The key is to work backwards from the last customer. Since half the eggs plus half an egg was all the remaining eggs, half the eggs must be equal to half an egg. So the last customer took one egg. If we add half an egg to this, we get half the number of eggs before the second customer took his, so there must have been three eggs, and the second customer took two (half of 3 is 1½, plus ½ equals 2). Since the first customer left 3 eggs, 3½ eggs must be half the number of eggs when he arrived. So there were 7 eggs, and the first customer took 4 (half of 7 is 3½, plus ½ equals 4).

9   Five for $20 would be the correct average price if they had both contributed the same *value* of ties. In that case it would make sense to average how many ties you can buy for $20 (four from the first seller, six from the second). But in fact they both contributed the same *number* of ties, so we should average the cost of a tie. The first seller sells six ties for $30, the second six ties for $20. So the average price should be six ties for $25.

10 After a 20% price rise the cost is £2,400. Then after a 20% reduction the price is £1,920. The price rise is 20% of £2,000, or £400. But the price drop is 20% of the new price of £2,400, which is £480.

11 a) 77 b) 350 c) 11,900

12 If 80% = £160 then 1% = £2, so 100% = £200.

13 If 60% = £300 then 1% = 300/60 = 5, so 100% = £500.

14 a) £21,000 b) 6.25% c) 57,000 d) The 30% discount is better. Buy one, get one half price is two for the price of 1.5, or one for the price of 0.75, which is the same as a 25% discount.

15 a) both give a discount of £1,200 b) 20% c) £525

16 $4 = 4 \times (4 - 4) + 4$; $5 = (4 \times 4 + 4)/4$; $6 = 4 \times .4 + 4.4$;
$7 = 44/4 - 4$; $8 = 4 + 4.4 - .4$; $9 = 4/4 + 4 + 4$; $10 = 44/4.4$;
$11 = 4/.4 + 4/4$; $12 = (44 + 4)/4$; $13 = 4! - 44/4$;
$14 = 4 \times (4 - .4) - .4$; $15 = 44/4 + 4$; $16 = .4 \times (44 - 4)$;
$17 = 4/4 + 4 \times 4$; $18 = 44 \times .4 + .4$; $19 = 4! - 4 - 4/4$;
$20 = 4 \times (4/4 + 4)$; $21 = (4.4 + 4)/.4$; $22 = 44 \times \text{sqrt}(4)/4$;
$23 = (4 \times 4! - 4)/4$; $24 = 4 \times 4 + 4 + 4$; $25 = (4 \times 4! + 4)/4$;
$26 = 4/.4 + 4 \times 4$; $27 = 4 - 4/4 + 4!$; $28 = 44 - 4 \times 4$;
$29 = 4/.4/.4 + 4$; $30 = (4 + 4 + 4)/.4$; $31 = (4! + 4)/4 + 4!$;
$32 = 4 \times 4 + 4 \times 4$; $33 = (4 - .4)/.4 + 4!$; $34 = 44 - 4/.4$;
$35 = 44/4 + 4!$; $36 = 44 - 4 - 4$; $37 = (\text{sqrt}(4) + 4!)/\text{sqrt}(4) + 4!$;
$38 = 44 - 4!/4$; $39 = (4 \times 4 - .4)/.4$; $40 = 44\text{-sqrt}(4 \times 4)$;
$41 = (\text{sqrt}(4) + 4!)/.4 - 4!$; $42 = \text{sqrt}(4) + 44 - 4$;
$43 = 44 - 4/4$; $44 = 44.4 - .4$; $45 = 4/4 + 44$;
$46 = 44 - \text{sqrt}(4) + 4$; $47 = 4! + 4! - 4/4$; $48 = 4 \times (4 + 4 + 4)$;
$49 = (4! - 4.4)/.4$; $50 = 4!/4 + 44$

NUMBER TRAINING CHALLENGES

1 a) 60% b) 9/20 c) 0.24 d) 260%

2 a) 8.5 b) 40 c) 2 d) 80

3 a) neither b) both c) both

4 He must have spent

$$1 - \frac{1}{4} - \frac{1}{5} - \frac{1}{3} = \frac{60 - 15 - 12 - 20}{60} = \frac{13}{60}$$

of his life as an old man. Since this is 13 years, his total life must have been 60 years.

5 The key is to work backwards, not forwards. Since Connie ate 1/3 she must have left 2/3 behind. So 2/3 of the sweets is 40 sweets, and the 1/3 she ate must be 20. This means that there were

60 sweets when Connie arrived – which is the 2/3 that Bruce left behind. The 1/3 he ate must have been 30 sweets, and there were 90 when he started. And this is the 2/3 that Amy left behind, so the 1/3 she ate must have been 45 sweets – and the box had 135 sweets in it at the start.

6 a) 44 b) 40% c) 95

7 False. The first 5% rise takes 100 to 105. The second 5% is now 5% of 105, and takes 105 to 110.25. The third 5% is 5% of this value, and takes it to 115.7625. Thus the combined rise is 15.7625%. This is an illustration of the phenomenon of *compounding*.

8 4, 9, 7, 9, 20 giving DIGIT.

9 June has 30 days, August and December each have 31, so the total is 92.

10 a) 219 b) 114 c) 372 d) 105

Chapter 5

1 To get to the next square number you need to add an extra row and an extra column to the square. So to get from $4^2 = 16$ to 5^2 you add an extra row (of length 4), and an extra column (now of length 5), so $5^2 = 16 + 4 + 5 = 25$. To get to 6^2 you add a row of length 5 and a column of length 6, so $6^2 = 25 + 5 + 6 = 36$.

2 A square with an area of 16 also has a perimeter of 16: the only time when the area and perimeter are the same.

3 5, 12, 13

4 To get to the next triangular number you need to add one more row to the bottom of the triangle. So if we call $T_1 = 1$ the first triangular number, $T_2 = 3$ the second triangular number, etc., then $T_3 = T_2 + 3 = 3 + 3 = 6$. And $T_4 = T_3 + 4 = 6 + 4 = 10$.

5 The sum of two consecutive triangular numbers is a square number. So $T_2 + T_3 = 3^2(3 + 6 = 9)$, $T_3 + T_4 = 4^2(6 + 10 = 16)$. You can see this easily with the help of a diagram:

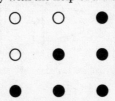

6

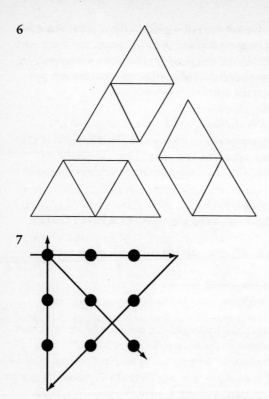

7

8 This is an example of perspective: two objects look the same size if one is twice as big but twice as far away. Imagine that the mirror is a window and your twin is standing on the other side: the image on the mirror is half as far away as the twin, so it's half the size.

mirror

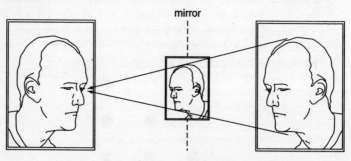

9 When made out of pieces bolted together, triangles are the only non-collapsible polygons.

10 There are an amazing 43, 252, 003, 274, 489, 856, 000 possible configurations of the Rubik's cube. How close was your educated guess?

NUMBER TRAINING CHALLENGES

1 A six-storey cannonball pile will have $1 + 3 + 6 + 10 + 15 + 21 = 56$ cannonballs.

3 First pull one end of the loop up the outside of your arm – inside the sleeve itself – then out at the top and over your head. Push it back into the top of your other sleeve and pull it down along the outside of the other arm, over your hand and back up the sleeve. At the top, pull it down inside the front of your jacket so that it comes down to your ankles – and you can climb out.

5 Imagine a line running from one corner to the opposite corner. Take a slice perpendicular to this line at the halfway point.

6 The central $1 \times 1 \times 1$ cube has six faces. Any cut can only reveal one of these faces, so six cuts are needed.

7 385

8 100

9 a) 979   b) 2,607   c) 54,472

10 Cut the cake into half, then each piece into half again with two normal cuts. Now cut each piece in half again with one horizontal cut. Of course, this only works if the cake doesn't have a nice topping!

Chapter 6

1 a) 1958   b) 1989   c) 1980   d) 1953

2 We opened up a standard tin and counted 411 beans.

3 Fill the three-litre container. Then fill the two-litre container from it. There will be one litre left over. Or, fill the two-litre container, and then empty it into the three-litre container. Fill the two-litre container again, and empty what you can into the three-litre container again. Since there's space for one more litre, one litre will be left in the two-litre container.

4

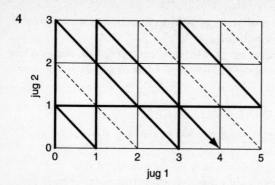

5 The average number of coins needed drops from 4.6 to 3.92.
6 If the circumference is C, the radius must be $C/2\pi$. Therefore the area must be
$$A = \pi \times (C/2\pi)^2 = C^2/4\pi.$$
7 Small: 63.62 in² for £6.95 is 10.9 pence per in².
Medium: 132.73 in² for £10.95 is 8.2 pence per in².
Large: 176.71 in² for £14.95 is 8.5 pence per in².
The medium is the best value.
8 a) 2 b) 6 c) 3

NUMBER TRAINING CHALLENGES

1 If you follow the obvious strategy and weigh four balls against four you'll narrow the heavier ball down to one of four balls. Weighing two of these against two narrows it down to one of two. Then you need a third weighing to determine which of these it is.

The key to reducing the number of weighings is to realize that you don't have to put all the balls on the scales in the first weighing. First weigh three balls against three balls. If these balance then the heavy ball must be one of the other two. Weigh them against each other to determine which it is. If the scales don't balance on the first weighing then you've narrowed down the heavy ball to one of three. Choose two of these balls to weigh against each other. If one side is heavier, that must be the heavier ball. If the scales balance, the third ball must be the heavier one.

3 55,000
4 Tip the barrel until the beer is just about to pour out. If the surface of the beer just touches the join between the sides and the base then the barrel is exactly half full, since the surface of the beer 'cuts' the barrel into two equal parts.

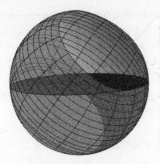

5 Rather than simply listing all the possible combinations of weights, you could use doubling to help. If you include the idea of a '0 g' weighing then each weight can either be on the scale or not. So each time you add a new weight, the number of weighing possibilities doubles: all the old possibilities without the new weight, and all the old possibilities with the new weight.

  ▷ With the 5 g weight you can weigh 0 g or 5 g (two possibilities).
  ▷ With 5 g and 10 g: 0 g or 5 g or 10 g or 15 g (four possibilities).
  ▷ With 5 g, 10 g and 20 g: 0 g or 5 g or 10 g or 15 g or 20 g or 25 g or 30 g or 35 g (eight possibilities).

So... with five weights there will be 32 possibilities – or 31 if you don't want to include '0 g' as one of them!

6 Here are the answers, correct to two decimal places. How close did you get?
  a) 40.64   b) 44.09   c) 18.18   d) 100,000,000
7 141 lengths (with 2 cm left over)
8 83.25 litres
9 1767 cm²
10 If the radius of a ball is R, then the height of the container is $6R$, while the circumference of the rim is $2\pi R$. Since π is more than 3, the circumference of the rim must be larger.

Chapter 7

1 There are many ways to explain the Monty Hall problem. The simplest way is to see that the chance you were right first time is 1/3. If you were wrong first time, then the prize is behind the other remaining door. So the chance of winning is 2/3 if you

switch. If this doesn't convince you, try the same trick but with a pack of playing cards (increasing the number of 'doors' from three to 52). You choose a card at random without looking at it. You'll win if you pick the ace of spades. If I examine the deck and show you 50 of the other cards, which are not the ace of spades, leaving one card in my hand… would you like to swap your card for the card I have now?

2

Total										
2	3	4	5	6	7	8	9	10	11	12
Number of ways to make it										
1	2	3	4	5	6	5	4	3	2	1
Probability										
1/36	1/18	1/12	1/9	5/36	1/6	5/36	1/9	1/12	1/18	1/36

3 You can think of this as tossing two coins, one to see if it rains on Saturday, and another to see if it rains on Sunday. There's a 25% chance that it rains on both days (HH), a 25% chance that it doesn't rain (TT), and a 50% chance that it rains on just one day (HT or TH).

4 The probability is 1/6 for the die multiplied by 1/2 for the coin, to give 1/12 overall.

5 a) There are three odd numbers out of six, so the chance of getting an odd number with the first die is 3/6 = 1/2. For the second die it's also 1/2, so the chance of getting a pair of odd numbers is 1/2 × 1/2 = 1/4.

   b) We want a head with the first OR a head with the second, so the probability is 1/2 + 1/2 − 1/4 = 3/4. Or we could say that the chance of getting at least one head is 1 minus the probability of getting no heads (ie getting two tails), which is 1 − 1/4 = 3/4. Or we could list the four possibilities (HH, HT, TH, TT) all equally likely, and note that in three out of the four we get at least one head.

   c) For the clothes to get soaked you need to have forgotten to take in the washing AND it needs to rain, so the probability is 0.2 × 0.5 = 0.1 or 10%.

   d) The chance of a history test is 1/10 or 0.1. The chance of a maths test is 1/5 or 0.2. So the chance of a history test OR a maths test is 0.1 + 0.2 − 0.02 = 0.28 or 28%. The chance of no test must be 72%. Maybe you calculated this faster by inverting the probabilities. The chance of no history test is 0.9. The chance of no maths test is 0.8. So, the chance of no history test AND no maths test is 0.9 × 0.8 = 0.72.

NUMBER TRAINING ANSWERS

1 Imagine turning cards over one after the other. The chance of the first being red is 5/7. Now there are four red cards left out of six, so the chance of the second also being red is 4/6. This leaves three red cards out of five, so the chance of the third also being red is 3/5. Altogether the chance of three reds is therefore 5/7 × 4/6 × 3/5, which comes to 2/7 – or just less than 29%. Although the chances of each card you turn over being red individually are all greater than 50%, the chance of them *all* being red is less than 50%, so it's not worth the bet.

2 The probability of winning is $\left(\frac{1}{6}\right)^6 = \frac{1}{46656}$
so the organizers would expect to have to give a car away once every 46,656 tickets. That means an income of £46,656 for every £12,000 spent on a car.

3 The probability of landing on red is 18/37 = 0.4865, so the expected return is 2 × 0.4865 = 0.973, which means you get on average 97.3p back for every £1 bet.

4 a) Every other number from the first onwards decreases by two, at the same time as every other number from the second increases by three. So the sequence continues 9, 11, 7...

 b) Here, the numbers of the Fibonacci sequence provide the increments: so, from 10, the numbers increase by 1, 1, 2, 3, 5, 8, 13... meaning that the next numbers in this particular sequence are 64, 98 and 153.

 c) 26 stands for the 26th letter of the alphabet, *z*, for *zero*. The 15th letter is *o* for *one*. *Two* starts with *t*, the 20th letter... and so on. To continue the sequence, *eight* begins with *e*, letter number 5; the *n* for *nine* is letter number 14; and *t* for *ten* gives you 20.

5 The chance of the dealer's second card being a picture card is 16/52 = 0.3077. So the expected return on an insurance bet is 3 × 0.3077 = 0.923, corresponding to a house edge of 7.7%.

6 With six non-picture cards already out of the deck, the chance that the dealer's remaining card is a picture card is 16/46 = 0.3478. In this case, the expected return on insurance is

$3 \times 0.3478 = 1.043$, or a player's edge of 4.3%. In this situation, insurance is definitely a good bet.

7

9	6	3	18
4	17	10	5
16	1	8	11
7	12	15	2

8 At first sight it seems that there are four possibilities for the buttons: all white, two whites and a black, two blacks and a white, and all black. Since two of these are all the same colour, you might be tempted to think that it's a 50% chance. But not all the possibilities occur with the same frequency. Since each button has two sides, and there are three buttons, there are really eight possible ways the buttons can land: WWW, WWB, WBW, WBB, BWW, BWB, BBW, BBB. Of these eight possibilities, only two have one colour showing. So the chances of winning are 2 in 8, or 1 in 4. This means that fair odds would be 3 to 1.

9 a) 55000 b) 614 c) 26 d) 138.44

10 The barman has the edge here, so it's probably not worth the risk. The probability that the first card is not a queen is 4/6. The probability that the second is also not a queen is 3/5 (since one card has been removed). So the probability that neither is a queen is

$$\frac{4}{6} \times \frac{3}{5} = \frac{2}{5}.$$

The chance that at least one is a queen is 3/5, or 60%.

Chapter 8

1 Let the ages be x and y. Then $x + y = 18$. $xy = 80$.
2 Let there be b boys and g girls. Then $b - 1 = g$. $b = 2(g - 1)$.
3 Let apples cost A and oranges cost O. Then $3A + 4O = 41$. $4A + 3O = 36$.
4 Let the total bill be T, and the individual contributions be A, B, and C (in pounds). Then $A + B + C = T$. Also $T/3 = A - 0.73$, and $T/3 = B + 0.37$. Finally $A = 10$.
5 $2x = 20$

6 $x + 3 = 8$

7 $x = 3$

8 $x = 3$

9 $x = 9 - y$

10 $3x - 21$

11 $S = D/T, T = D/S$

12 $16 = 4x.$

13 Doubling the first equation gives $4y = 20 - 8x$. Substituting into the second equation gives $-5x + 20 = 15$. Solving for x gives $x = 1$, so $y = 3$.

14 The formula for bricks is: $b = 2n + 2$. So animal 10 will have 22 bricks in its body, and animal 1,000 will have 2,002.

15 Let the rate of working be R widgets/man/hour. Then, with M men producing W widgets in T hours,

$$R = \frac{W}{M \times T} = \frac{20}{5 \times 2} = 2$$

and, rearranging the formula,

a) $M = \dfrac{W}{R \times T} = \dfrac{14}{2 \times 1} = 7$

b) $T = \dfrac{W}{R \times M} = \dfrac{12}{2 \times 8} = \dfrac{3}{4}$

c) $W = R \times M \times T = 2 \times 3 \times 5 = 30$

18 $7x + 5 = 3x - 25$

$7x - 3x = -25 - 5$

$4x = -30$

$x = -30/4$

$x = -15/2$

19 $5x - (3x - 1) = x - 4$

$5x - 3x + 1 = x - 4$

$2x - x = -4 - 1$

$x = -5$

NUMBER TRAINING CHALLENGES

1 We have $A = 4B$. Also $(A + 10) = 3(B + 10) = 3B + 30$. Substituting for A gives $4B + 10 = 3B + 30$. Collecting terms gives $B = 20$. So $A = 80$.

2 60 cm. The logical solution looks like this:

$x = 30 + (x/2)$

$2x = 60 + x$

$x = 60$

3 Look closely at the 'proof'. There's a step where you're dividing both sides of the equation by x, and this is the 'naughty step'. x is zero, so you're not allowed to divide by it.

4 We are told that $A_{now} = 2 B_{then}$, $A_{then} = B_{now}$, $A_{now} - B_{now} = 5$, and $A_{now} - A_{then} = B_{now} - B_{then}$. Rearranging and eliminating gives
$A_{now} - A_{then} = B_{now} - B_{then} = 2 B_{then} - B_{now}$,
so that $B_{now} = 3/2 \, B_{then}$. Since $A_{now} = 2 B_{then}$ we must have
$2 B_{then} - 3/2 \, B_{then} = 5$, so that $B_{then} = 10$, $B_{now} = 15$, $A_{then} = 15$, $A_{now} = 20$.
When Ben is 20, Amy will be 25.

5 Let's assume that the Earth is a sphere. If we call its radius R and the initial length of the rope – the circumference – C, then we can show how the circumference relates to the radius:
$C = 2\pi R$.

Increasing the length of the rope by one means that C goes to $(C + 1)$ and we want to know what the change in R is, so let's say that R goes to R + r. Since the rope still forms a circle, we must have
$C + 1 = 2\pi(R + r) = 2\pi R + 2\pi r = C + 2\pi r$.

Cancelling the C from each side gives

$$r = \frac{1}{2\pi} \approx 0.16.$$

So the rope is about 16 cm off the ground everywhere along its length!

6 My friend put down two £1 coins, so it was clear he wanted to pay £2 for a double scoop. I, on the other hand, put down a single £2 coin, and the man behind the counter didn't know if I was expecting to get £1 change.

7 Two thousand fish would be a good estimate. If you call the number of fish in the lake F, then the proportion of tagged fish in the lake is 100/F. The proportion of tagged fish in the second sample was 5/100. If you assume that this is the same as the proportion of tagged fish in the lake, then

$$\frac{5}{100} = \frac{100}{F}.$$

A bit of rearrangement gives

$$F = \frac{100 \times 100}{5} = 2000.$$

8 a) 180   b) 803   c) −256   d) 2162

9 Add five lines to spell N I N E.

10 You can solve this problem with the equation: $3(100,000 + x) = 10x + 1$

(Adding 100,000 puts a 1 at the front of a five-digit number, and multiplying by ten and adding one puts a 1 at the end of a number.) Solving this gives:

$$10x + 1 = 3(100,000 + x)$$
$$10x + 1 = 300,000 + 3x$$
$$10x = 299,999 + 3x$$
$$7x = 299,999$$
$$x = 299,999/7 = 42,857$$

So the answer is 42,857.

Chapter 9

1 Continuing this sequence, going up three bases each time, the result will continue to be less than 20 in the corresponding base notation – and here's why. For each new number in the sequence you're effectively adding four. Since the base is increasing by three each time, the '1' is worth three extra in the new base, so to add four you only need to add 1 to the units column, and the sequence looks very normal: 12, 13, 14, etc. It's tempting to think that after 19 you'd get to 20; but remember: when you write $4 \times 12 = 19$ you're actually in base 39, so the '1' in that answer is worth 39. Next you'd be trying to write 4×13 (52) in base 42: a 1 in the '42s' column, and then... you've got a problem! You want to show 10 in the units column. To write this number – and indeed to use bases greater than ten in general – you need a single digit presentation for the number ten. Computer programmers sometimes use base 16 – 'hexadecimal' – and they write the letters A to F to represent the numbers ten to 15. In that case Alice's numbers would proceed 1A, 1B, etc. Since the bases used are getting higher and higher she needs more and more symbols as the numbers progress. In base 42, for example, she's going to need a single digit representation for all the numbers from zero to 41. And since the base is always larger than the number in the units column (the base is going up by three each time, the units by one), she will never, ever get to 20.

2 The Pigeon's false logic is an example of the following argument: 'All dogs have four legs. My cat has four legs. Therefore my cat is a dog.' A similar argument is often used by politicians: Something must be done. This is something. Therefore this must be done. To refute the Pigeon you'd have to point out that the fact that all serpents eat eggs does not imply that all egg-eating beings are serpents.

NUMBER TRAINING CHALLENGES

1 Each move reduces the number of sections by one. There are 1,000 sections to start with. There's one section at the end. So, it takes 999 moves, no matter what order the moves are made in.

2 Neither of the statements necessarily follows. The facts here would be true if all women drank coffee and no men drank coffee.

3 A quick method would be to work in from both 'ends', pairing numbers to make 100. $0 + 100 = 100$, $1 + 99 = 100$, $2 + 98 = 100$, $3 + 97 = 100$, etc. until you got to $49 + 51 = 100$. That's 50 lots of 100, 5,000, plus the 50 in the middle: 5,050.

4 a) 11 (you might have said that 10% is 5.5, so 20% = $5.5 + 5.5 = 11$) b) 12 (75% of 16) c) 49 (10% + 5% + 2.5% = $28 + 14 + 7$) d) 20 (1% is 2.5 and $2.5 \times 8 = 20$)

5 The mathematically-minded manager knows that the discounts need to be applied successively. This is exactly the same as the compounding of interest. Let's say the meal costs £100. The first discount is 25% of 100, and takes the cost to £75. The second discount is now 35% of 75 (not 35% of 100), taking the cost down to £48.75. The final discount is 40% of 48.75, reducing the cost of the meal to £29.25 – and giving a total discount of 70.75%.

6 This is just the jigsaw problem in disguise. Each match eliminates one player. We start with 117 players, and we finish with one champion, so we need to hold 116 matches.

7 Call the length of the head H, body B and tail T. You know that

$$T = H + \frac{B}{4}.$$

$$B = \frac{3}{4}(T + B + H).$$

$$H = 4.$$

Multiplying both sides of the first two equations by four, and replacing H with its known value of four, gives you

$$4T = 16 + B.$$

$$4B = 3B + 3T + 12.$$

So...

$4T = 16 + B = 16 + 3T + 12 = 3T + 28$.

Subtracting $3T$ from each side gives $T = 28$, revealing that $B = 3T + 12 = 96$. So the total length of the fish is $4 + 96 + 28 = 128$ inches.

8 You could use the letters M and W for the number of men and women in the town. The number of married men is $0.3M$ and the number of married women is $0.4W$. Since the number of married men must equal the number of married women, $0.3M = 0.4W$, so $W = 0.75M$. The total number of people in the town is $M + W = M + 0.75M = 1.75M$. Of these, $0.7M$ are single men, so the fraction of single men is $0.7/1.75$, which is 0.4: 40%.

9 The third digit after the decimal point is 1, the fifth is 9, the seventh is 6.

10 Yes and no. It depends on what you mean by *on average*. The average number of legs of people in the UK is less than two: nobody has more than two legs, but a few people have fewer than two legs. But *on average* is also used colloquially to mean *in the norm*, in which case it would be asking for the most common occurrence (this is another statistic used to analyse data, called the *mode* in mathematics). The most common number of legs is two.

Chapter 10

1 a) $1.234567 \times 10^6 \approx 1.23 \times 10^6$
    b) $5.656123676 \times 10^9 \approx 5.66 \times 10^9$
    c) $9.3790003984833 \times 10^{10} \approx 9.38 \times 10^{10}$

2 a) 3.9×10^{-4} b) 6.07008×10^{-5} c) 1.101001×10^{-7}

3 Accepted wisdom used to be that it was impossible to fold a sheet of paper in half more than seven or eight times, no matter what size the sheet of paper, because the paper becomes too thick to fold. However, in 2002 an American high school student successfully folded a special 4,000 ft roll of toilet paper 12 times (it took her and her family seven hours to do it!). In 2006, the TV show *Mythbusters* attempted to beat this record by folding taped-together sheets the size of a football field in half (turning 90 degrees each time) with the help of steam rollers and fork lift trucks, but they only managed 11 folds.

NUMBER TRAINING CHALLENGES

1 There are many ways to solve this problem. One way is to ask either of the men which way the *other* man would direct you. No matter who you ask, he will point out the wrong way to go, so you simply take the other path. An alternative approach is to say to either man: 'If I were to ask you which way to go, which way would you direct me?' The truth teller will simply point to the correct path. The liar *would* have pointed to the wrong path if you'd just asked him that, but in answer to your actual question he'll also point to the correct path.

2 a) 5.67×10^6 b) 4.7654532×10^3 c) 1.23×10^{-9}
  d) $4.354312398225 \times 10^{10}$

3 The key to logic problems like this is to work backwards from the end. If only one pirate is left he will get all the money. So, if there are two pirates left, number 1 will always vote against number 2 no matter how many coins he's offered, since that way he gets to keep all the money and kill a pirate. Since number 2 needs a clear majority to win, he's doomed. And pirates 1 and 2 know that if it gets down to the last 2, number 2 will die and number 1 will get all the money.

Now suppose there are three pirates left. Number 1 will again vote against, since if the proposal is turned down then he will get all the money and kill two pirates. Number 2 will always vote for any proposal by number 3, because otherwise he's doomed to die. So number 3 can keep all the money, and the proposal will be passed by 2 votes to 1 (because he's bound to vote for his own proposal). If it gets down to three pirates left, then number 3 gets 100, and numbers 1 and 2 get 0.

Suppose there are four pirates left. Number 4 needs two of the others to support him. Number 3 will never support him, since by defeating the proposal he can gain the whole 100 coins. But number 4 can gain the support of numbers 1 and 2 by offering just 1 coin each. After all, if the proposal is defeated, they'll get nothing. So number 4 keeps 98 and gives one each to numbers 1 and 2, and nothing to number 3.

Now we can work out what to do if we're the fifth pirate. We need two of the others to support us. The cheapest way to get this support is to offer one to number 3 (who otherwise will receive nothing), and two to number 1 (or number 2). There is no need to offer number 4 or number 2 anything, and we get to keep 97 of the coins ourselves!

4 Yes, it's true; and we can use proof by contradiction to show it. Suppose there is a prime number p greater than three, which is not one more or one less than a multiple of six. This means p is not of the form $6n + 1$ or $6n + 5$, where n is a whole number. Then p must be of the form $6n$, $6n + 2$, $6n + 3$, or $6n + 4$. But $6n$, $6n + 2$ and $6n + 4$ are divisible by 2, while $6n + 3$ is divisible by 3. This contradicts the fact that p is a prime number.

5 101: 'One hundred and one'.

6

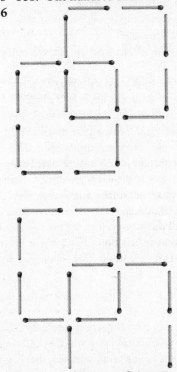

7 All the digits are in alphabetical order.

8 18

9 The key piece of information appears right at the beginning of the puzzle: 'Imagine you're driving a bus from the coast to the city'.

10 1

Test yourself now

1 a) 20 b) 65
2 a) hello b) igloo c) hillbillies
3 North West
4 d) 100
5 22, 12, 4, 9, 11 = E, O, W, R, P = POWER
6 a) 3 b) ∞ c) $x - a$
7 a) 68 b) 77 c) 22 d) 473
8 If $a = x$ (as in the first line of the 'proof') then $(a - x) = 0$ so we are not allowed to divide by it (as in the last line).
9 Since I have no brothers, my father's son is me. Therefore I am that man's father. So that man is my son.
10 False. The facts are consistent with all the mathematicians being men, for example.
11 Suppose your friend chose the number a. Multiplying by ten gives $10 \times a$. Subtracting a gives $9 \times a$. Dividing by a gives 9. So no matter what number your friend chose, by this stage the number on their calculator screen is 9. Now squaring gives 81, and adding 19 gives 100. Now suppose your number is n. The next number you ask them to subtract is $100 - n$. This leaves $100 - (100 - n) = n$.
12 If you have a thin rectangular box, measuring 4 ft by 3 ft, then the pole will fit nicely along the diagonal.
13 $123 - 45 - 67 + 89 = 100$
14

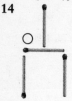

Index

Numbers are filed as they are spelled.

Notes

Notes

Notes

Notes

Notes

Notes

Notes

Notes